Orthognathic Surgery

Orthognathic Surgery
A Synopsis of Basic Principles and Surgical Techniques

George Dimitroulis, MDSc (Melb.), FDSRCS (Eng.), FFDRCS (Irl.)
Clinical Fellow in Oral and Maxillofacial Surgery
University of Florida College of Dentistry
Gainesville, Florida, USA

M. Franklin Dolwick DMD, PhD
Assistant Dean for Hospital Affairs
University of Florida College of Dentistry
Gainesville, Florida, USA

Joseph E. Van Sickels DDS
Director of Graduate Education
Department of Oral and Maxillofacial Surgery
University of Texas Health Science Center at San Antonio
San Antonio, Texas, USA

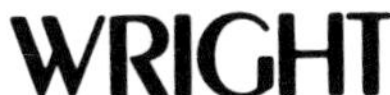

Wright
An imprint of Butterworth-Heinemann Ltd
Linacre House, Jordan Hill, Oxford OX2 8DP

A member of the Reed Elsevier plc group

OXFORD LONDON BOSTON
MUNICH NEW DELHI SINGAPORE SYDNEY
TOKYO TORONTO WELLINGTON

First published 1994

British Library Cataloguing in Publication Data
Dimitroulis, George
Orthognathic Surgery: Synopsis of Basic Principles and Surgical Techniques
I. Title
617.52059

ISBN 0 7236 1017 7

Typeset by Keytec Typesetting Ltd, Bridport, Dorset
Printed and bound in Great Britain by Biddles Ltd, Guildford and King's Lynn

Contents

Preface

Orthognathic surgery has incredibly expanded the scope of oral and maxillofacial surgery over the last few decades. It has become an important fundamental skill that is acquired in most oral and maxillofacial surgical training programmes worldwide. Since it is also a surgical field that few surgeons outside the dental profession understand or practise, it is vital that all present and future oral and maxillofacial surgeons establish a firm grasp of the fundamental concepts behind the principles and practice of this somewhat difficult and complex area of surgery.

Surgical training invariably involves a large clinical commitment which not surprisingly leaves precious little time for the surgical trainee to devote to reading through the enormous volumes of textbooks and journals. The broad and concise overview contained in this small handbook will hopefully prove to be quite popular as a useful means of preparation for seminars, lectures, conferences and examinations.

The book is not meant to replace any of the larger texts in the field of orthognathic surgery, but rather, to complement them. Indeed, the assumption is made that the student or clinician who would be attracted to this book would already have some background of the principles, clinical aspects and management of dentofacial deformities. Each chapter presents a broad outline containing only the very 'meat' of the subject that has been trimmed of all the excess 'fat' so that a basis can be rapidly established for further reading in this constantly growing field of surgery.

GM
MFD
JEVS

Chapter 1

Introduction

Orthognathic surgery

In its simplest definition, orthognathic surgery refers to the 'alignment of the jaws'. Hence the aim of orthognathic surgery is to normalize the relationship of the jaws between themselves and to the rest of the craniofacial complex. Successful treatment of dentofacial deformities with orthognathic surgery depends on a thorough understanding of dental occlusion, facial growth, functional gnathology and facial aesthetics.

Facial growth

Intrauterine development

1. *Ovum* 0–8 days
2. *Embryo*

    a. Presomite 8–20 days
    b. Somite 21–31 days – flat disc to tube with somites
    c. Postsomite 4–8 weeks – *rapid growth of organs and tissues, and period during which the orofacial complex first becomes recognizable as a distinct entity*

3. *Foetus* 3 months–term – rapid growth but little organogenesis or tissue differentiation

Orofacial development (*Fig. 1.1*)

Orofacial development is genetically predetermined so that discrepancies between tooth–jaw size, shape and morphology will readily reflect the orofacial form and pattern of the parents. Occasionally dentofacial deformities such as cleft lip and palate may be the result of environmental insults to the developing embryo which may occur during crucial stages or periods of

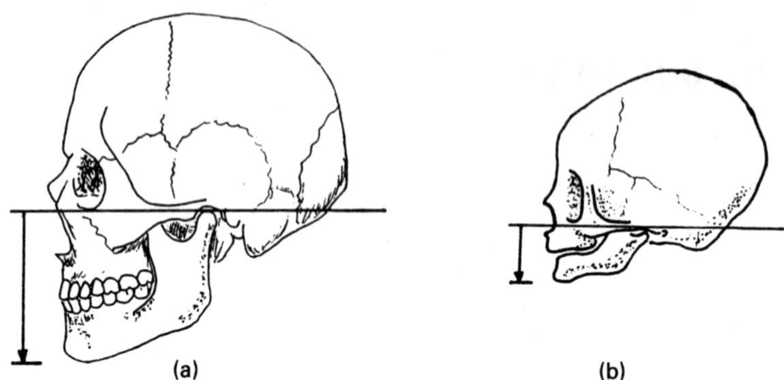

Figure 1.1 Comparative sizes of facial skeletons relative to cranium in an adult (a) and infant (b).

gestation. Generally speaking, less than 10% of a given population will have dentofacial deformities that may benefit significantly from orthognathic surgery.

Theories of dynamic skeletal growth processes

1. Growth movements

    a. Cortical drift
    b. **Displacement**

2. Remodelling
3. Relocation
4. Rotation
5. V-principle

Displacement theories

1. *Sutural growth* (Sicher)
   Growth of the skull was largely intrinsic and the control fell equally between cartilage, sutures and periosteum. Growth of the skull bones was therefore independent of adjacent structures.
2. *Nasal septum theory* (Scott)
   Skeletal growth was largely determined by cartilagenous 'growth centres' which possessed intrinsic control.
3. *Functional matrix theory* (Melvin Moss)
   Osseous growth of the skull is entirely secondary to the growth

and functional demands of the soft tissues of the head and neck. This is the most acceptable theory at present.

Functional matrix theory

1. Each functional cranial component consists of two parts:

    a. *A functional matrix* – all soft tissues and functional spaces
    b. *A skeletal unit* – all the osseous, cartilagenous and tendonous tissues which protect and support the specifically related functional matrix

2. The growth of the functional matrix is controlled by its neural innervation, thus growth is ultimately controlled by higher neural centres (neurotrophism)
3. The skeletal units have NO direct genetic predetermination and exist only to protect and support their related functional matrix (excepting homeostatic functions). Therefore the growth of a skeletal unit is ALWAYS secondary to the primary growth of its related functional matrix. As the soft tissue capsule expands, the bones become passively translated in space which is in turn compensated by growth at the sutural margins and cartilagenous areas which are hence secondary growth areas. Examples:

    a. The existence and dimensions of alveolar bone is entirely influenced and dependent upon the presence, size and position of the teeth
    b. The coronoid process only exists to serve as a functional attachment of the temporalis muscle to the mandible

The effects of surgery on facial growth

Orthognathic surgery must be tailored to the growth pattern of each individual. Importantly, it must consider the growth potential of the patient and target those regions where growth is undesirable. It is generally unknown to what degree surgery affects subsequent facial growth. From studies on cleft patients, the degree of restricted growth after surgery appears to depend on the stage of development of the child at the time of the primary surgery and the amount of tissue manipulation and subsequent scarring that takes place. There are two phases where orthognathic surgery may be undertaken:

1. *During the growth phase* – otherwise considered as *interceptive surgery*, whereby surgery is used to restrict unfavourable growth (*growth which is detrimental to the child's health and psychosocial wellbeing and development*) so as to minimize the degree of the subsequent dentofacial deformity. Usually, but not always, a second surgical procedure may be required at the end of the growth phase
2. *After growth has ceased* – in adulthood, whereby orthognathic surgery may be considered as *definitive surgery*

Controversy exists as to whether some deformities can be treated early and others only after growth is complete. It is not uncommon, for example, to operate on a mandibular horizontal deficiency during early adolescence, while a mandibular horizontal excess case will not be treated until well after growth is complete.

Common dentofacial deformities (*Fig. 1.2*)

In the classification of dentofacial deformities, it is preferable to describe the skeletal relationship rather than simply the dental relationships, since orthognathic surgery is fundamentally used to correct the underlying skeletal base discrepancies.

Maxillary deformities

Maxillary anteroposterior (AP) excess

Protrusive maxilla where there is an overgrowth in an anterior horizontal direction. There is often a class II molar relationship, sometimes combined with mandibular protrusion (bimaxillary protrusion).

Maxillary AP deficiency (*Fig. 1.2a*)

Inadequate growth of the maxilla in an anterior direction with a class III malocclusion.

Vertical maxillary excess (*Fig. 1.2b*)

Overgrowth of the maxillary alveolus in the inferior direction creating excess tooth and gingival display and often associated with an incompetent lip seal without mentalis muscle strain.

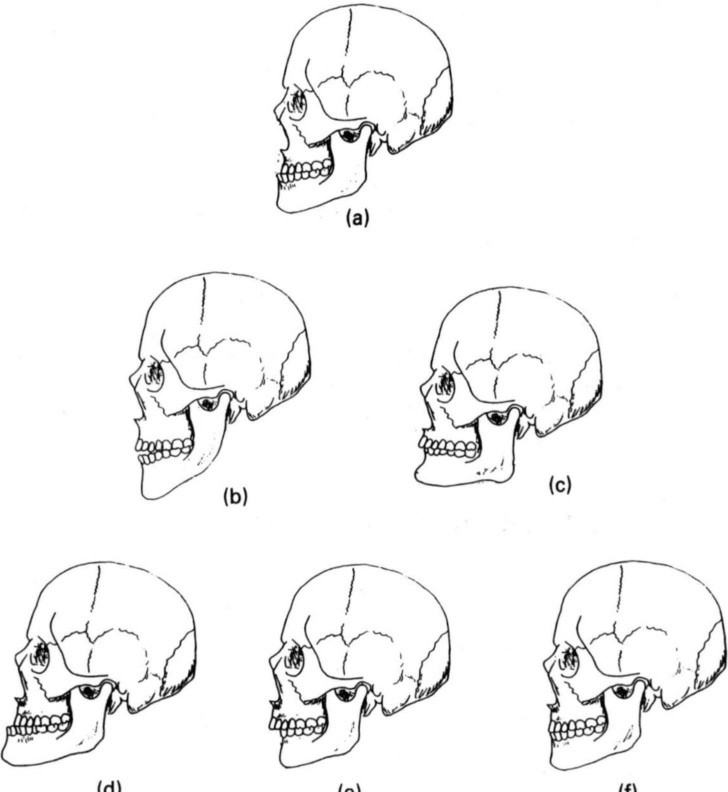

Figure 1.2 Common dentofacial deformities. (a) Maxillary AP deficiency. (b) Vertical maxillary excess with anterior open bite – dolicofacial. (c) Vertical maxillary deficiency with deep overbite – brachyfacial. (d) Mandibular AP excess. (e) Mandibular AP deficiency. (f) Normal skeletal profile.

Vertical maxillary deficiency (Fig. 1.2c)

Edentulous appearance showing no teeth, often combined with a deep bite in the mandible and prominent 'chin button'. Short lower face.

Alveolar clefts

Usually present with maxillary constriction in AP and transverse dimensions.

Mandibular deformities

Mandibular AP excess (hyperplasia) (*Fig. 1.2d*)

Prognathism with class III malocclusion.

Mandibular AP deficiency (hypoplasia) (*Fig. 1.2e*)

Deficient anterior growth of mandible with class II malocclusion.

Mandibular asymmetry

Usually related to unbalanced excess or lack of growth on one side of the mandible, often the condylar process, but sometimes the ramus and body may be involved. Malocclusion may or may not be present depending on any compensatory growth in the maxilla which may or may not have occurred. Clinically appears as a chin and mandibular midline shift (lower facial asymmetry).

Chin deformities

Often associated with other mandibular deformities.

Macrogenia

Overgrowth of chin in vertical or anterior direction.

Microgenia

Chin deficiency in vertical and/or anterior direction.

Combined maxillary–mandibular deformities

Short face syndrome (*Fig. 1.2c*)

Brachyfacial – deficient lower facial growth in the vertical dimension. Low mandibular and occlusal plane angles. Usually class II malocclusion with mandibular AP deficiency, but sometimes combined with vertical maxillary deficiency.

Long face syndrome (*Fig. 1.2b*)

Dolicofacial – excess lower facial height usually with increased occlusal and mandibular plane angles. Often a combination of vertical maxillary excess and mandibular hypoplasia.

Apertognathia (*Fig. 1.2b*)

Anterior open bite. Often associated with long face syndrome or simply increased posterior facial height.

Lower facial asymmetry

Usually caused by unbalanced aberrant growth in the mandible, e.g. condylar hyperplasia. Alteration in the maxillary cant will only arise if problem emerges during normal facial growth, whereby compensatory growth of the maxilla will occur in relation to the aberrant mandibular growth pattern.

Uncommon dentofacial deformities

These are often associated with rare craniofacial syndromes (see Chapter 11)

Cleft lip and palate

1. Pierre Robin syndrome
2. Treacher-Collins syndrome (otomandibulofacial dysostosis)
3. Apert's syndrome

Facial asymmetry

1. Hemifacial atrophy (Parry–Romberg syndrome)
2. Hemifacial microsomia (Goldenhar syndrome)
3. Hemifacial hypertrophy
4. Neurofibromatosis (von Recklinghausen's disease)

Midface deficiencies

1. Craniosynostoses

    a. Apert's
    b. Crouzon's
    c. Pfeiffer

2. Binder's syndrome
3. Achondroplasia dwarf
4. Cleidocranial dysplasia

Mandibular deficiencies

1. Pierre Robin syndrome
2. Treacher-Collins syndrome (otomandibulofacial dysostosis)
3. Hemifacial microsomia (Goldenhar syndrome)

Mandibular prognathism

1. Gorlin–Goltz syndrome
2. Osteogenesis imperfecta
3. Marfan syndrome
4. Klinefelter syndrome

Further reading

Bachmayer D, Ross B and Munro I (1986) Maxillary growth following LeFort III advancement surgery in Crouzon, Apert and Pfeiffer syndromes. *Am. J. Orthod.* **90**, 420.

Bell WH, Proffit WR and White PR (1980) *Surgical Correction of Dentofacial Deformities*. Vols 1 and 2. WB Saunders, Philadelphia.

Bell WH, Proffit WR and White PR (1985) *Surgical Correction of Dentofacial Deformities.* Vol 3. WB Saunders, Philadelphia.

Bishara SE and Thorp RM (1977) Effects of Von Langebeck palatoplasty on facial growth. *Angle Orthod.* **47**, 34.

Enlow DH (1990) *Facial Growth*. 3rd ed. WB Saunders, Philadelphia.

Epker BN and Wolford LM (1980) *Dentofacial Deformities*. CV Mosby, St Louis.

Gorlin RJ, Cohen MM and Levin LS (1990) *Syndromes of the Head and Neck*. 3rd ed. Oxford University Press, Oxford.

McNamara J (1982) *Effect of Surgical Intervention on Craniofacial Growth*. Ann Arbor, University of Michigan, Center for Human Growth and Development.

Moss ML (1968) The primacy of functional matrices in orofacial growth. *Dent. Pract.* **19**, 65.

Moss ML (1969) The primary role of functional matrices in facial growth. *Am. J. Orthod.* **55**, 566.

Nanda R, Sugawara J and Topazian R (1983) Effect of maxillary osteotomy on subsequent craniofacial growth in adolescent monkeys. *Am. J. Orthod.* **83**, 391.

Proffit WR and White RP (1991) *Surgical–Orthodontic Treatment*. Mosby Year Book, St Louis.

Schumacher GH (1985) Factors influencing craniofacial growth. *Prog. Clin. Biol. Res.* **187**, 3.

Scott JH (1953) The cartilage of the nasal septum. *Br. Dent. J.* **95**, 37.

Shapiro P *et al*. (1981) The effects of early LeFort I osteotomies on craniofacial growth of juvenile macaca monkeys. *Am. J. Orthod.* **79**, 492.

Sicher H (1947) The growth of the mandible. *Am. J. Orthod.* **33**, 30.

Sperber GH (1989) *Craniofacial Embryology*. [4th edn.] Wright, London.

Chapter 2

Orthognathic planning

Introduction

Philosophy of orthognathic planning

1. Obtain a functional occlusion with teeth in most ideal position to aid stability and aesthetics
2. Correct underlying skeletal disharmony
3. A surgical plan with a maximum aesthetic result that does not compromise occlusal or skeletal stability

Objectives

Must strike an optimal balance between:

1. Aesthetics
2. Function
3. Stability

Aesthetics should not be sacrificed at the expense of function and indeed in most instances, an improvement in function will bring about an improvement in aesthetics.

Patient evaluation and diagnosis

Gathering diagnostic information involves:

1. *Patient concerns* – to determine the patients' feelings about the existing problems and their expectations for treatment results
2. *Clinical evaluation*

    a. Facial form – frontal and profile
    Long, short, convex, concave, flat
    b. Relationship of facial thirds (*Figs 2.1* and *2.2*)
    Proportional: middle vs lower, long, short

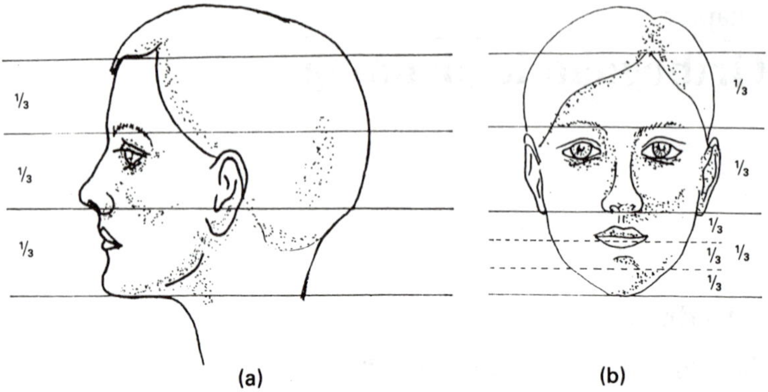

(a) (b)

Figure 2.1 Proportional relationship of facial thirds. (a) Profile. (b) Full face.

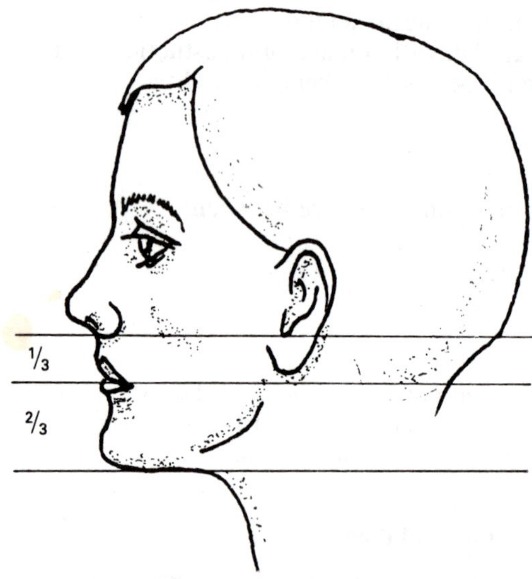

Figure 2.2 Lower facial proportions, upper lip to lower lip 1:2.

c. Relationship of soft tissues to dentition
   Smile line, occlusal cant, dental midlines vs soft tissues
d. Clinical measurements (*Figs 2.2* and *2.3*)

   i. Vertical dimensions
   ii. Anteroposterior dimensions
   iii. Transverse dimensions
   iv. Intra-arch dimensions

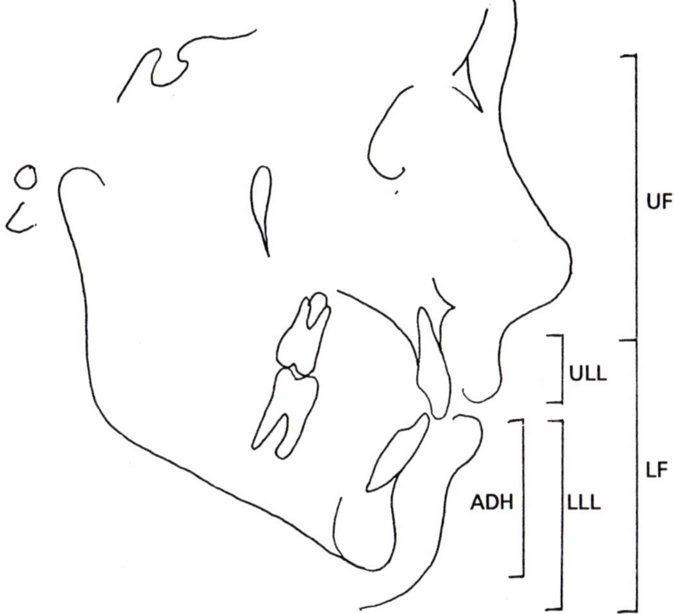

Figure 2.3 Vertical facial dimensions. ADH, anterior dental height (40–44 mm). ULL, upper lip length (20–22 mm). LLL, lower lip length (44–52 mm). UF, upper face height to (LF) lower face height 5:6.

3. *Radiographic analysis* (*Figs 2.4–2.6*)

   a. Cephalometric – lateral and antero-posterior
      Lips must be in repose, teeth only lightly touching and in centric relation
   b. Orthopantomogram – check for position of inferior alveolar canal and screen for gross pathology

4. *Dental study models*

   a. Accurate bite registration – facebow indicated in two jaw surgery
   b. Two jaw cases require duplicate models

   Note – trimmed or mounted models should match the degree of discrepancy seen in the lateral cephalogram

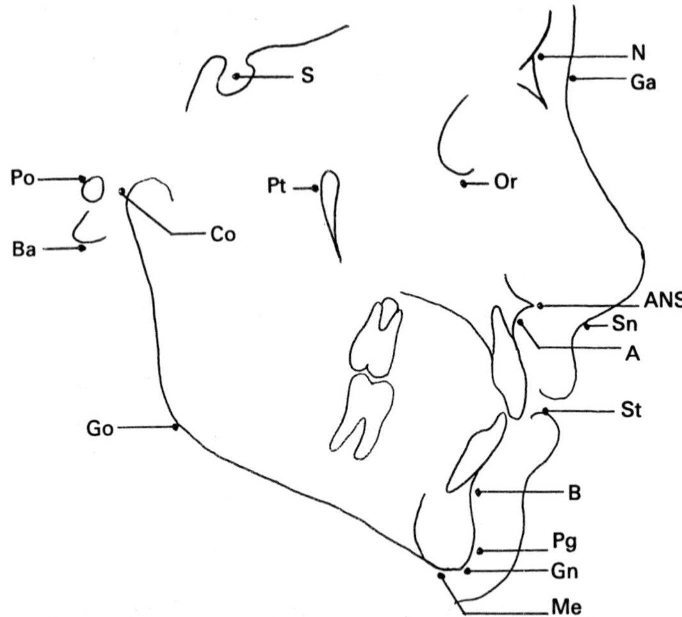

Figure 2.4 Some important cephalometric points. Po, porion; Ba, basion; Go, gonion; Co, condylonium; Pt, pterion; S, sella; Or, orbitali, N, nasion; Ga, glabella; ANS, anterior nasal spine; Sn, subnasali; A, A point; St, stomion, B, B point, Pg, pogonion; Gn, gnathion; Me, menton.

5. *Other*

   a. Speech
   b. Audiometry
   c. Psychological
   d. Medical

Sequence of treatment planning

1. Dental and periodontal treatment
2. Extractions
3. Presurgical orthodontics
4. Orthognathic surgery
5. Postsurgical orthodontics
6. Definitive general dental management and maintenance
7. Other, e.g. rhinoplasty

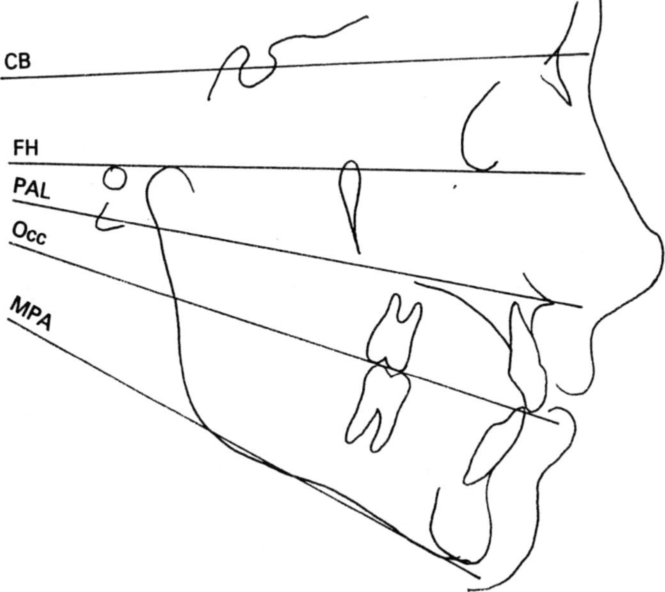

Figure 2.5 Horizontal facial planes. CB, cranial base; FH, Frankfurt horizontal; PAL, palatal plane; Occ, occlusal plane angle relative to FH = 8 ± 4°; MPA, mandibular plane angle relative to FH = 25 ± 4°.

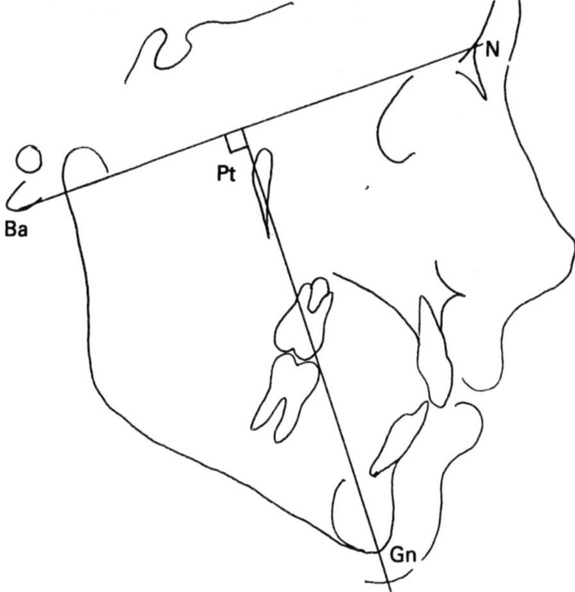

Figure 2.6 Facial axis = 90°.

Patient evaluation

Clinical evaluation

Patient positioning

- Patient should be standing with head oriented so that Frankfurt horizontal is parallel to floor, i.e. natural head position
- Mandible in centric relation with condyles properly seated in fossae
- Teeth lightly touching together
- Lips should be relaxed and not forced together

Facial thirds (*Fig. 2.1*)

1. Upper third – forehead
2. Middle third – between the eyebrows and base of nose
3. Lower third – from the base of the nose to the undersurface of the chin

Frontal view

- Intercanthal distance = alar base width (28–34 mm)
- Dental vs soft tissue midlines (chin, nose, upper lip) – to assess facial asymmetry
- Lip lengths: upper = 22 ± 2 mm, lower = 40–44 mm (*Fig. 2.2*)
- Upper central incisal display at rest = 2–4 mm
- Gingival display at rest and when smiling
- Vermillion display, i.e. overclosure increases lower vermillion display

Lateral view

- Glabella to base of nose = base of nose to soft tissue chin
- Relationship of globe to surrounding tissues
- Lower lip length = 2 × upper lip length (*Fig. 2.2*)
- Chin–throat angle
- Nasal tip–upper lip angle
- Labiomental fold and lip competence

Oral examination

- Teeth in centric relation and occlusion
- Intra-arch

1. Crowding, tipped, missing, decayed or rotated teeth
2. Curve of Spee
3. Periodontal health
4. Curve of Wilson – buccal tilting of posterior teeth

- Interarch

1. Occlusion, molar and canine relationships
2. Transverse discrepancies – crossbites
3. Overbite, overjet, midline shifts
4. Freeway space

Radiographic analysis (STO)

The *surgical treatment objective* (STO) is a visual projection of the changes in skeletal, dental and soft tissues as a result of surgical–orthodontic treatment. According to Wolford *et al.* (1985) the STO was designed as both a diagnostic aid and a treatment planning aid and hence developed to:

1. Present a simple and accurate method of predicting results of surgical orthodontic treatment
2. Establish the surgical movements necessary to correct the deformity
3. Accurately predict the resultant facial profile
4. Provide a visual aid with a single overlay

Initial STO

Prepared before commencement of treatment to determine the orthodontic and surgical goals.

Final STO

Prepared before surgery to determine the exact vertical and horizontal skeletal and soft tissue changes to be achieved.

Radiographic guidelines suggested by Wolford et al. (1985)

1. Upper tooth to upper lip relationship (1–4 mm)
2. Upper lip length = 20–22 mm (*Fig. 2.2*)
3. Vertical bony height of face (upper:lower = 5:6 ratio) (*Fig. 2.3*)
4. Lower anterior dental height (40–44 mm) (*Fig. 2.3*)
5. Maxillary depth (FH to NA = 90°) (*Fig. 2.7a*)

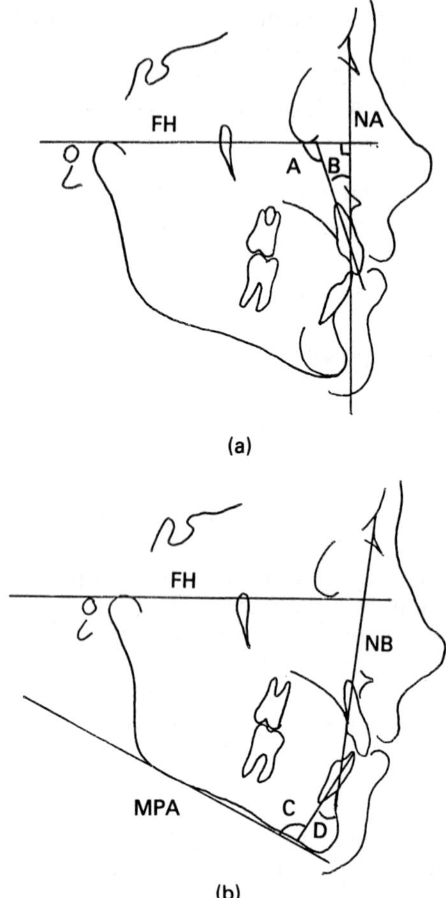

Figure 2.7 Incisor inclinations. (a) Upper incisor angulation. Angle A: 112° relative to FH. Angle B: 22° relative to NA with incisor tip 4 mm in front of NA. (b) Lower incisor angulation. Angle C: about 90° to MPA. Angle D: 20° relative to NB with incisor tip 4 mm in front of NB.

6. Mandibular plane angle to FH (25°) (*Fig. 2.5*)
7. Mandibular depth (FH to NB = 88°) (*Fig. 2.7b*)
8. Occlusal plane angle (8° ± 4) (*Fig. 2.5*)
9. Soft tissue thickness (lip – upper and lower, chin = 1:1:1) (see Chapter 3)
10. Upper incisor angulation (to NA = 22°, incisor tip = 4 mm in front of NA) (*Fig. 2.7a*)
11. Lower incisor angulation (to NB = 20°) (*Fig. 2.7b*)

Dental model analysis

There are ten basic aspects that should be analysed:

1. Arch length – room to fit all teeth in line of arch
2. Tooth size analysis – *Bolton's index* total width of six upper anterior teeth = 1.3 × total width of lower six anterior teeth
3. Tooth position
4. Arch width analysis – assess transverse problems
5. Curve of Spee
6. Cuspid–molar position
7. Overbite/overjet relationship
8. Tooth arch symmetry – comparing left and right symmetry within each arch
9. Buccal tooth tip
10. Missing, broken-down or crowned teeth

Treatment planning

Dental and periodontal treatment

The objective is to maintain as many of the teeth as possible and to stabilize the periodontium prior to orthodontic and surgical intervention.

Extractions

1. To facilitate orthodontics, i.e. bicuspids
2. To facilitate subsequent surgery – lower third molars extracted 9–12 months prior to sagittal split osteotomy otherwise there will be a weakened lingual cortex

Presurgical orthodontics

Different dentofacial patterns respond very differently to treatment (see Chapter 6).

Brachyfacial (short face). Flat mandibular plane where growth tends to proceed horizontally. Best to use a non-extraction technique.

Dolicofacial (long face). Steep mandibular plane angle. Growth tends to proceed vertically. More likely to use extraction technique.

Where skeletal form is unfavourable, dentoalveolar segments will compensate. Therefore, most of these dental compensations must be corrected prior to surgery, by positioning teeth in their ideal axial relationship to their respective skeletal bases.

Primary goals of presurgical orthodontics

1. Position the teeth over their respective basal bone
2. Align and level the teeth
3. Adjust for tooth size discrepancies
4. Correct rotated teeth
5. Divergence of roots adjacent to surgical sites
6. Co-ordination of upper and lower arch widths – correct transverse discrepancies without compromising stability and dental health, otherwise must consider further surgical options (see later)

Surgery

Surgery is designed to reposition the basal bone and/or dento-alveolar segments into more normal interrelationships. The aim is to provide the best functional and aesthetic result and provide stability of the achieved results.

Surgical preparation

1. Final STO tracing (*Fig. 2.8*)
2. Model surgery and occlusal wafer

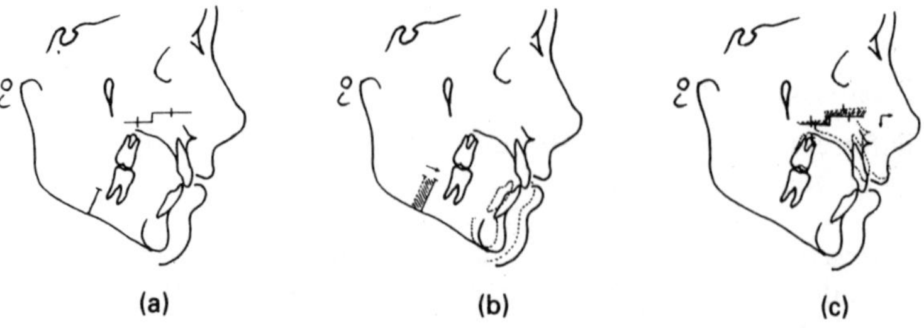

Figure 2.8 Surgical treatment objectives planned on cephalometric tracings. (a) Surgical reference lines for maxilla and mandible. (b) Planning for mandibular advancement surgery. (c) Planning for maxillary advancement and downgraft surgery.

Postsurgical orthodontics

May take up to 10 months to fine tune the final occlusion whilst the bones and muscles continue to heal and adapt to the repositioning, depending on the accuracy of the preoperative set-up of the occlusion.

Objectives

1. Final tooth alignment and root parallelism
2. Maximal interdigitation
3. Ideal overbite and overjet
4. Centric occlusion = centric relation

If rigid fixation is used, orthodontics can resume anywhere from 2 to 6 weeks postsurgery whereby the teeth and osseous segments can move very rapidly during the first few months postop, hence the orthodontist should initially see patient on frequent basis (every 1–2 weeks) for adjustments so rapid changes can be closely monitored. A good presurgical orthodontic set-up will help to simplify the surgery, improve the result in terms of stability and occlusion, and decrease the amount of postsurgical orthodontics required.

Further reading

Barnett DP (1975) Variations in the soft tissue profile and their relevance to the clinical assessment of skeletal pattern. *Br. J. Orthod.* **2**, 235.

Bell R, Kiyak H *et al*. (1985) Perceptions of facial profile and their influence on the decision to undergo orthognathic surgery. *Am. J. Orthod.* **88**, 323.

Broch J, Slagsvold O and Rosler M (1981) Error in landmark identification in lateral radiographic headplates. *Eur. J. Orthod.* **3**, 9.

Burstone CJ (1967) Lip posture and its significance in treatment planning. *Am. J. Orthod.* **53**, 262.

Epker BN and Fish LC (1986) *Dentofacial Deformities: Integrated Orthodontic and Surgical Correction.* CV Mosby, St Louis.

Epker BN and Wolford LM (1980) *Dentofacial Deformities*. CV Mosby, St Louis.

Powell N and Humphreys B (1984) *Proportions of the Aesthetic Face.* Thieme-Stratton, New York.

Precious D and Delaire J (1987) Balanced facial growth: a schematic interpretation. *Oral Surg. Oral Med. Oral Pathol.* **63**, 637.

Proffit WR and White RP (1991) *Surgical–Orthodontic Treatment*. Mosby Year Book, St Louis.

Ricketts RM, Schulhof RJ and Bagha L (1976) Orientation: sella-nasion or Frankfurt horizontal. *Am. J. Orthod.* **69**, 648.

Shah SM and Joshi MR (1978) An assessment of asymmetry in the normal craniofacial complex. *Angle Orthod.* **48**, 141.

Wolford LM, Hilliard FW and Dugan DJ (1985) *Surgical Treatment Objectives: A Systematic Approach to the Prediction Tracing.* CV Mosby, St Louis.

Chapter 3

Genioplasty

Introduction

Genioplasty is used to describe the numerous surgical techniques used to alter the size and morphology of the bony chin with concomitant changes in the surrounding soft tissues. Otherwise known as mentoplasty, chin surgery is commonly combined with other orthognathic procedures. About 15% of all dentofacial deformities primarily involve the chin.

Historical

In the past, most surgical chin procedures involved the use of alloplastic implants for augmentation. In 1942, Hofer described the osteotomy of the anterior lower border of the mandible via an extraoral submental incision. Later, in 1957, Trauner and Obwegeser described the intraoral approach, or labial sulcus incision, to the osteotomy of the anterior mandibular lower border.

Applied anatomy

The chin is a region of the lower face consisting of bone and soft tissue elements. The bony chin is basically the mental protruberance bounded by the mental tubercles superiorly, mental foramenae laterally and the lower border of the anterior mandible inferiorly. In surgery, the most important structures to keep in mind are:

1. *Mental nerves (foramen)* – major sensory innervation of the chin
2. *Mentalis muscles* – indirectly provide the major vertical support to the lower lip in addition to chin posture
3. *Lingual muscle pedicle* – provides the major blood supply to the osteotomized segment of the chin, hence maintains viability of the bone and prevents resorption

4. *Root apices of lower incisors* – must identify root apices and design osteotomy cuts at least 5 mm below these

Chin deformities

These may be aesthetic (e.g. macrogenia) or functional (e.g. chin ptosis). Chin deformities may occur in isolation, but are more commonly associated with other dentofacial deformities.

Functional deformities (commonly iatrogenic)

1. Chin ptosis
2. Lower lip incompetence

Aesthetic deformities

1. Macrogenia (large chin)
   a. Vertical
   b. Horizontal (anteroposterior)
   c. Combination of a and b
2. Microgenia (small chin)
   a. Vertical
   b. Horizontal (anteroposterior)
   c. Combination of a and b
3. Asymmetry

Evaluation of the chin

1. Clinical

a. Lip competence
b. Lower lip length:upper lip length (approx 2:1) (*Fig. 3.1a*)
c. Position of chin point in relation to midline facial axis (symmetry)
d. Labiomental fold
e. Chin–throat angle
f. Mentalis muscle strain

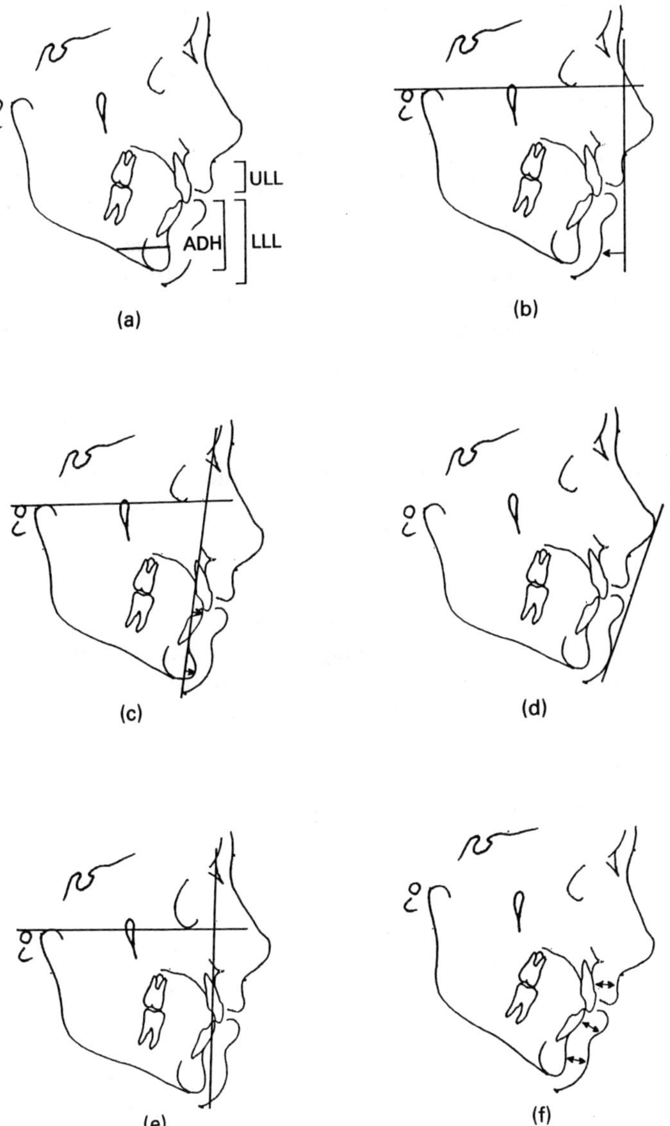

Figure 3.1 Cephalometric evaluation of the chin. (a) Vertical proportions of lower face ULL:ADH = 1:2. (b) Subnasali perpendicular. (c) NB line to chin projection. (d) Aesthetic S-line. (e) McNamara perpendicular. (f) Soft tissue thickness.

2. Cephalometric (*Fig. 3.1*)

a. Anterior dental height – 40 mm females, 44 mm males (approx mean) (*Fig. 3.1a*)
b. Frankfurt horizontal – subnasali perpendicular (0–3 mm posterior for soft tissues) (*Fig. 3.1b*)
c. Anterior projection from NB line – should equal projection of lower incisor (approx 4 mm) (*Fig. 3.1c*)
d. S-line – chin to nasal tip should have lips in balance. (*Fig. 3.1d*)
e. McNamara perpendicular (FH–nasion perpendicular) – pogonion should be on or close to this reference line (*Fig. 3.1e*)
f. Soft tissue thickness – upper lip:lower lip:chin = 1:1:1 (*Fig. 3.1f*)

3. According to sex

Males tend to prefer a strong chin prominence whereas females tend to opt for less chin.

4. Soft tissue changes

These are difficult to predict but recently reported as 1 to 0.9 ratio of bone to soft tissue changes for advancement genioplasty. Movements in other directions more controversial since most reports are of short-term follow-up studies.

Basic principles of genioplasty

1. Approach

a. Submental–semilunar incision which follows lingual border of anterior mandible
   Provides good access, particularly for adjunctive procedures such as submental lipectomy (see Chapter 9)
b. Labial sulcus – incision placed 1 cm forward of the sulcus depth

2. Dissection

a. Transection of mentalis muscle
b. Expose, isolate and protect mental nerves bilaterally
c. Maintain soft tissue attachment at the inferior border

3. Horizontal osteotomy

a. Made at least 5 mm below the root apices of lower incisors
b. There are numerous osteotomy designs

Genioplasty osteotomy designs

i. Horizontal – most commonly used (*Fig. 3.2a*)
ii. Double horizontal – for large advancements

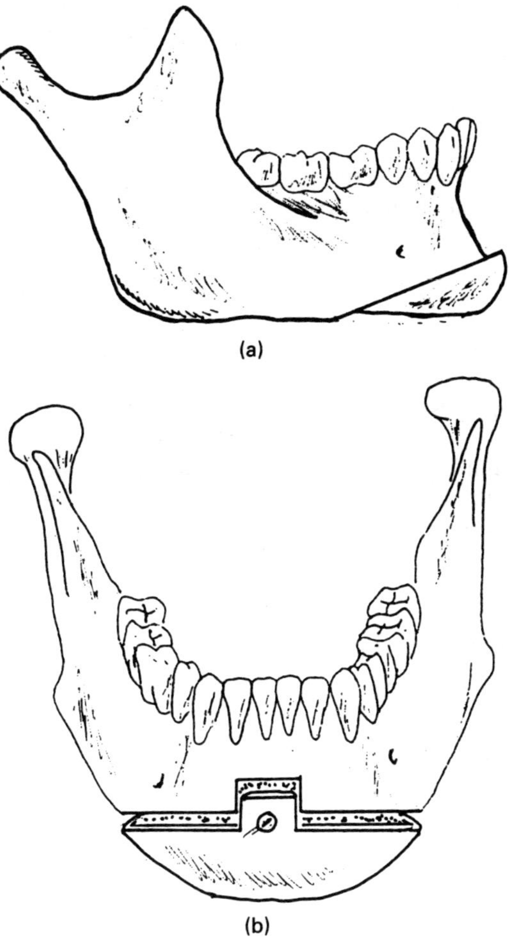

Figure 3.2 Genioplasty techniques. (a) Simple horizontal sliding advancement. (b) Tenon–Mortise procedure for vertical changes.

iii. Tenon–Mortise (*Fig. 3.2b*)
iv. Sagittal (Thompson 1985)
v. Horizontal–vertical step osteotomies

4. Down-fracture and repositioning

a. Must always maintain an attached broad based lingual muscle pedicle to the osteotomized bony chin segment
b. By virtue of its simple anatomy and surgical versatility, the osteotomized chin may be repositioned in any three dimensions or directions, viz horizontal, lateral or vertical planes

5. Fixation

a. Transosseous wires
b. Bone plates and screws
c. Lag screws

6. Closure

a. Must restore mentalis muscle continuity
b. Close in two layers
c. Light pressure dressing

Note. Chin implants are placed in a subperiosteal pocket and are often not fixed by any means apart from surrounding soft tissue pressure which holds them in place.

Genioplasty techniques

Functional genioplasty

First described by Michelet in early 1970s. Used to correct abnormal mentalis muscle activity at an early age by surgically altering the underlying bone chin deformity.

Indications

1. Vertical chin excess – requiring vertical reduction genioplasty
2. Horizontal (anteroposterior) chin deficiency – requiring advancement genioplasty

Timing

Usually undertaken just after the eruption of the lower canines.

Augmentation genioplasty

1. Alloplastic onlay grafts – various materials including hydroxylapatite (see Chapter 8)
2. Biological onlay grafting – allogenic or autogenous bone (prone to resorption)
3. Horizontal advancement osteotomy (*Fig. 3.2a*)
4. Vertical downgraft osteotomy with interpostional graft
5. Lateral expansion – midline osteotomy with outward rotation of the genial segments

Reduction genioplasty

1. Shave (osteoplasty) of chin protruberance – high incidence of ptosis
2. Horizontal sliding osteotomy and setback
3. Vertical reduction osteotomy with wedge ostectomy (bone removal)
4. Lateral reduction – with midline ostectomy for broad based chins

Asymmetrical genioplasty

Asymmetrical vertical shift of genial segment (propellor type genioplasty).

Complications of genioplasty

1. Mental nerve paraesthesia/anaesthesia

   a. Excessive stretching or retraction intraoperatively
   b. Direct injury to nerve

2. Chin ptosis

   a. If mentalis muscle is totally stripped off bone and not reattached

3. Lower lip incompetence

   a. When mentalis muscle is totally stripped off bone and not reattached
   b. Poor placement of incision site
   c. Poor primary closure resulting in excessive scarring

4. Poor aesthetics – double chinning effect caused by reduction genioplasty in thick necks
5. Resorption

   a. Of bone underlying alloplastic chin implant
   b. Of bony chin especially where lingual muscle pedicle is stripped off

6. Necrosis – of bony chin especially where it is completely denuded of all soft tissue attachment
7. Dislodgement – of osteotomized bone segment or migration of onlay graft
8. Haematoma, infection, wound dehiscence

   a. Poor surgical technique
   b. Stripping off periosteal envelope from inferior border

9. Relapse – which is related to:

   a. Degree of advancement – large advancements more likely to relapse. Role of suprahyoid musculature may be an important factor
   b. Fixation – rigid fixation more stable than wire osteosynthesis for small to moderate advancements
   c. Bone resorption (see 5 above)

10. Periodontal defects and abnormal frenum arise when incision is made too close to the attached gingivae

Further reading

Bell WH (1985) Genioplasty strategies. In: Bell WH (ed): *Surgical Correction of Dentofacial Deformities: New Concepts*. Vol 3, pp 57–70. WB Saunders, Philadelphia.

Bell WH and Gallagher DM (1983) The versatility of genioplasty using a broad pedicle. *J. Oral Maxillofac. Surg.* **41**, 763.

Ellis E, Dechow PC, McNamara JA *et al*. (1984) Advancement genioplasty with and without soft tissue pedicle: An experimental investigation. *J. Oral Maxillofac. Surg.* **42**, 637.

Epker BN and Fish LC (1986) *Dentofacial Deformities: Integrated Orthodontic–Surgical correction*. CV Mosby, St Louis.

Epker BN and Wolford LM (1980) *Dentofacial Deformities*. CV Mosby, St Louis.

Hinds EC and Kent JN (1969) Genioplasty: the versatility of horizontal osteotomy. *J. Oral Surg.* **37**, 690.

Hofer O (1942) Operation der Prognathie und Mikrogenie. *Dtsch. Zahn. Mund. Kieferheilk.* **9**, 121.

Hohl TH and Epker BN (1976) Macrogenia: a study of treatment results with surgical recommendations. *Oral Surg.* **41**, 545.

Polido WD, Regis LDC and Bell WH (1991) Bone resorption, stability and soft tissue changes following large chin advancements. *J. Oral Maxillofac. Surg.* **49**, 251.

Rubens BC and West RA (1989) Ptosis of the chin and lip incompetence: consequences of lost mentalis muscle support. *J. Oral Maxillofac. Surg.* **47**, 359.

Schendel SA (1985) Genioplasty: a physiologic approach. *Ann. Plast. Surg.* **14**, 506.

Thompson ERE (1985) Sagittal genioplasty: a new technique of genioplasty. *Br. J. Plast. Surg.* **38**, 70.

Trauner R and Obwegeser HL (1957) The surgical correction of mandibular prognathism and retrognathia with consideration of genioplasty. *Oral Surg.* **10**, 677.

Wolford LM, Hilliard FW and Dugan DJ (1985) *Surgical Treatment Objectives: A Systematic Approach to the Prediction Tracing*. CV Mosby, St Louis.

Zide BM and McCarthy J (1989) The mentalis muscle: an essential component of the chin and lower lip position. *Plast. Reconstr. Surg.* **83**, 413.

Chapter 4

Mandibular surgery

Introduction

Orthognathic procedures of the mandible are classified according to the design of the osteotomy and the region where the surgery is undertaken, i.e. body or ramus. Osteotomy refers to bone cuts, whereas ostectomy involves the removal of bone.

Classification

Ramus procedures

1. Condylotomy (subcondylar osteotomy)
2. Condylectomy
3. Sagittal split
4. Vertical subsigmoid
5. Inverted 'L'.
6. 'C' or arcing osteotomy
7. Postcondylar grafts

Body procedures

1. Anterior to mental foramen

    a. Step osteotomy/ostectomy
    b. Midline symphyseal

2. Posterior to mental foramen

    a. Y-ostectomy
    b. Rectangular ostectomy
    c. Trapeziod ostectomy
    d. Inverted 'V' ostectomy

3. Mandibuloplasty

Subapical body procedures

1. Anterior

    a. Kole
    b. Combined with midline symphyseal

2. Posterior
3. Total

Genioplasty

See Chapter 3.

Ramus procedures

Where large movements of the mandible are necessary, i.e. whole dental arch.

Condylotomy (subcondylar osteotomy)

Indications

Condylar neck is sectioned to correct mild mandibular prognathism. Occasionally used to treat TMJ internal derangement.

Approaches

1. Extraoral – retromandibular, submandibular
2. Intraoral – most common approach
3. Blind – Gigli saw, of historical interest only

Extraoral

- Condylar neck is sectioned obliquely and mandible repositioned posteriorly
- Simple overlap of condylar neck is all that is required for union

Intraoral (transoral)

- Poor access mandates special retractors in condylar region
- Variations of the condylar or subcondylar osteotomy have been suggested to facilitate condylar placement

- The condylar head should remain in fossa and the neck fragment should overlap the ramus of the mandible on its lateral aspect
- MMF = 6 weeks, although some authors suggest shorter period

Blind approach

- First described by Kostecka in 1931. Later reviewed by Ward (1961) and Banks and MacKenzie (1975)
- Risks – damage to facial nerve and mandibular nerve. Unpredictable haemorrhage from maxillary vessels.
- Not in the current standards of practice; of historical interest only

Condylectomy

Indications (see Chapter 7)

1. Ankylosis
2. Tumours, e.g. osteochondroma
3. Condylar hyperplasia
4. Mandibular asymmetry
    a. Hemifacial microsomia
    b. Unilateral mandibular
        i. Hypertrophy
        ii. Elongation

Surgical technique

- Preauricular incision, sometimes with temporal extension for greater access
- Horizontal osteotomy through the neck of the condyle made at predetermined level. Deepest portion of bone (medially) sectioned with an osteotome
- After lateral pterygoid muscle and joint capsule is stripped away, condyle fragment is mobilized and removed. Capsule is primarily closed with insertion of drain tube and firm pressure dressing applied postoperatively
- Further orthognathic surgery should be postponed 3–9 months

Fixation

- Not required for small shifts
- Training elastics (MMF) required for more extensive shifts
- For immediate joint reconstructions MMF is required until callous begins to form in 5–7 days

PA cephalometric measurements

Required to determine the amount of condylar head to be excised and calculate the increase in height of condyle by measuring from gonion to bimastoid line.

Combined with other procedures

- Immediate or delayed joint reconstruction
- Other mandibular or maxillary osteotomies

Sagittal split osteotomy

The most versatile mandibular osteotomy.

Historical review (*Fig. 4.1*)

Trauner and Obwegeser (1957) (Fig. 4.1a). Horizontal cut just above mandibular foramen on medial side of ramus. Vertical cut taken down anterior border of ramus. Oblique cut made through lateral cortex towards angle of jaw. Good technique for mandibular set-back but poor bone contact with mandibular advancement. Aseptic necrosis of angle due to extensive stripping of the pterygomasseteric sling.

Dalpont (1961) (*Fig. 4.1b*). Modified the sagittal split by advancing the oblique cut towards the molar region and making the vertical cut through the lateral cortex. The main problem with set-backs was interference between main retropositioned proximal fragment and the mastoid process where occasional pressure on the facial nerve may occur as well.

Hunsuck (1968) (*Fig. 4.1c*). Shortened the cut through the medial cortex of the ramus by taking it only as far as the mandibular foramen which prevented the occasional shattering of the ramus in mandibular set-backs.

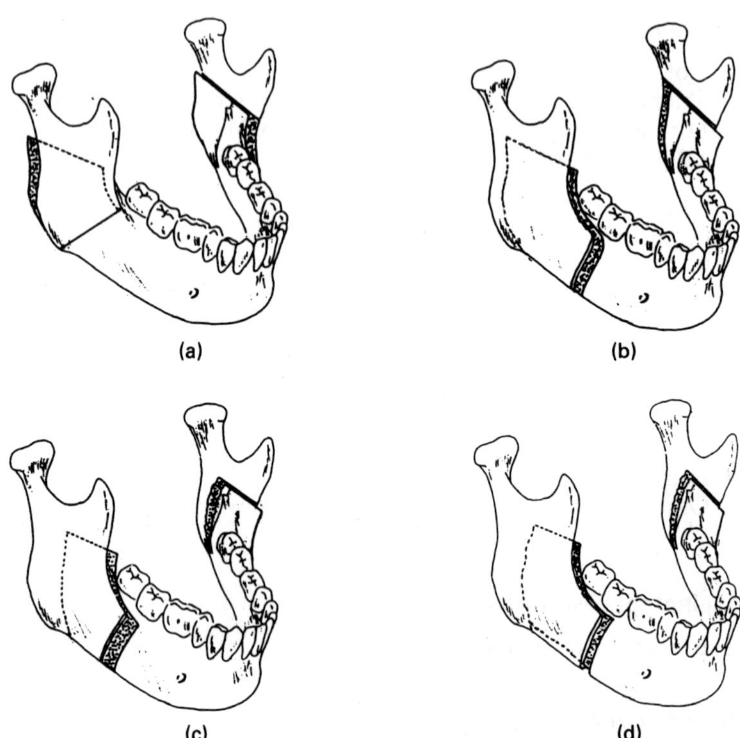

Figure 4.1 Evolution of the sagittal split ramus osteotomy. (a) Original Trauner and Obwegeser (1957). (b) Dalpont modification (1961). (c) Hunsuck modification (1968). (d) Bell and Schendel, Epker *et al*. modification (1977–78).

Bell and Schendel (1977) and Epker et al. (1978) (*Fig. 4.1d*). In the anterior vertical cut, the whole of the lower border is sectioned through and through. The split is kept more laterally by directing fine osteotomes down the inner surface of the lateral cortex to produce easier splitting and greater protection for the inferior dental nerve. Blood supply to the ramus is preserved as elimination of need to strip the pterygomasseteric sling.

Surgical technique

Incision. Lateral crest of alveolus. Extended up the anterior border of ramus and anteriorly along external oblique ridge as far forward as first or second molar.

Dissection. Subperiosteal exposure laterally over body of mandible to lower border. Medially just beyond the lingula and superiorly to expose the coronoid process.

Osteotomy

1. Lingual cortex of ramus – from anterior border of ramus, passing backwards to just reach superiorly and posteriorly to lingula
2. External oblique ridge – cuts made down along anterior border of ramus, medial to external oblique ridge then forwards to about the 2nd molar tooth
3. Vertical cut – lateral cortex of the body down to and through lower border of mandible

Split. Begin from lower border of vertical cut then proceed to insert fine osteotomes along alveolar cut to gently pry the two fragments apart. The neurovascular bundle must always lie on medial side in the distal segment otherwise it should be repositioned there.

Fixation options (see Chapter 8)

1. Upper border transosseous wires – 4–6 week period of intermaxillary fixation required
2. Lower border transosseous wire – 4–6 week period of intermaxillary fixation required
3. Bicortical screws – inserted transbuccally via trochar and cannula or transorally in an oblique fashion in selected cases. Best biomechanical advantage is obtained with three screws placed in a triangulation pattern
4. Monocortical plates and screws – one or two plates may be used and often placed transorally

Postoperative

- Drain tubes are optional and often unnecessary
- Wire fixation – MMF for 6 weeks
- Screw fixation – training elastics for few days

Note:

- Relapse is more likely to occur if there is rotational movement of the proximal fragment particularly with set-backs

- To prevent relapse in mandibular setback procedures the medial pterygoid muscle attachment may be partially stripped off
- Occasionally the sphenomandibular ligament prevents large advancement of the mandible and may need to be stripped off the lingula
- For large advancements (> 8 mm) additional measures such as skeletal suspension wires should be considered even when rigid internal fixation is used

Limitations of the sagittal split procedure

1. Relapse is common in cases of:

   a. Anterior open bite – not appropriate to use sagittal split alone particularly with short ramus height, where the inverted 'L' osteotomy is better suited. Sagittal split may be used in conjunction with maxillary osteotomy
   b. Mandibular asymmetry – rotatory movements predispose to poor contact between the fragments hence careful trimming minimizes angle flaring

2. Thin/abnormal ramus structure – better to use inverted 'L', 'C' or arcing osteotomies
3. Split is occasionally unpredictable

Vertical subsigmoid (or ramus) osteotomy (VSS) (*Fig. 4.2a*)

Developed by Caldwell and Letterman (1954).

1. Mainly for set-back procedures and mandibular asymmetries
2. Not recommended for correction of anterior open bites

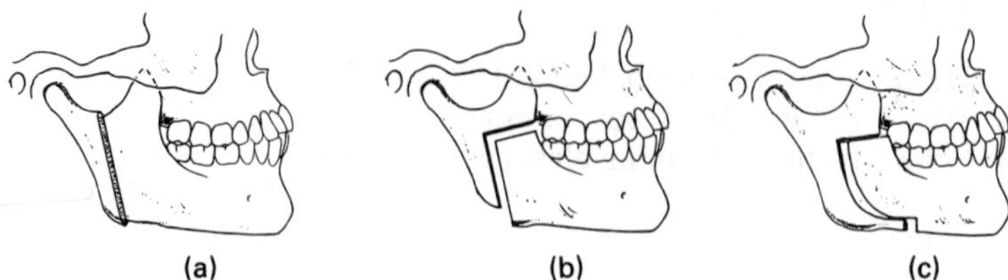

Figure 4.2 Variations of mandibular ramus osteotomies. (a) Vertical ramus (subsigmoid) osteotomy. (b) Inverted 'L' osteotomy. (c) 'C'-shaped osteotomy.

Extraoral approach (for unusual cases only)

1. Easiest and safest method is to utilize Risdon (submandibular) approach
2. Whole lateral surface of ramus is stripped of periosteum and masseter muscle
3. Medial pterygoid muscle insertion is reflected off the deep surface
4. Rayne subsigmoid retractor with fibreoptic light attachment is inserted
5. Position of lingula identified by a small bony thickening on the lateral surface of the ramus. A vertical bone cut is made a few millimetres posterior to this landmark with a slight oblique angle anteroposteriorly
6. Mandible is set-back so that proximal fragment overlaps the distal fragment on the outer aspect. Lateral surface decortication may be required on the distal fragment to establish good bony contact and healing and on the proximal fragment to prevent deformity at the angle. Trimming of the angle from proximal fragment may also be necessary to prevent flaring. Transosseous fixation may or may not be used although Epker and Wolford (1980) advocate wiring to ensure the condyle is carefully seated in fossa
7. Where setbacks are greater than 1 cm, a coronoidectomy may be necessary so as to prevent excessive tension on temporalis muscle
8. Closure in layers – muscle, deep fascia, platysma and skin
9. MMF = 6 weeks

Disadvantages

a. External scar
b. Occasional damage to mandibular branch of facial nerve

Transoral approach

1. Has become a more popular approach since the introduction of specially designed retractors, oscillating saws, fibreoptic illumination, irrigation and suction
2. Submentovertex X-ray may occasionally help to assess the amount of outward flaring of the rami in order to establish feasibility of the transoral approach, since the more parallel the rami, the less direct vision available to the surgical sites
3. Extended 3rd molar incision up the anterior border of ascend-

ing ramus and forwards to 1st molar similar to the sagittal split osteotomy incision

4. Extensive muscle stripping from ramus may result in aseptic necrosis of bone fragment and condylar sag. However if inadequate muscle stripping occurs then there is an increased risk of relapse. Bell *et al*. (1980) recommend that medial pterygoid muscle should not be stripped off since it maintains the blood supply to the proximal fragment and helps keep condyle in place although some believe this leads to greater relapse
5. Osteotomy begins halfway, first up then down from sigmoid notch to angle using oscillating saw with 120° blade angle. Depth of cut should be no greater than 6 mm to avoid risk of damage to medial tissues

Inverted 'L' osteotomy (*Fig. 4.2b*)

Devised by Pichler and Trauner (1948).

Indications

1. For increasing height (length) of ramus which also requires an interpositional bone graft
2. Mandibular advancements
3. Mandibular set-backs – provided the proximal fragment is carefully trimmed back

Surgical technique

1. Submandibular approach similar to VSS but incision is made further down in the neck
2. *Vertical* cut made above and behind the lingula
3. *Horizontal* cut above lingula may be more easily executed via transoral approach

'C' osteotomy (*Fig. 4.2c*)

Modification of the inverted 'L' osteotomy devised by Caldwell *et al*. (1968).

Indications

Mandibular advancement in patients with a high mandibular plane angle often without the need for bone grafting although a defect remains posteriorly.

Surgical technique

1. Vertical cut is brought forwards just below the level of the inferior dental nerve in a horizontal direction towards the third molar tooth
2. Osteotomy is completed by making a short vertical cut anteriorly through the lower border
3. Fixed with lower border wiring or plates

Arcing osteotomy

Epker and Wolford (1980).

Window is cut in the region of the lingula. The inferior alveolar nerve is identified and the cut follows the canal in an anterior direction whilst preserving its contents.

Postcondylar grafts

Trauner (1954). Modified by Banks and Ardouin (1980).

Indications

- Not commonly used outside Britain
- Used as an early step in the management of severe mandibular retrusion so as to minimize the degree of advancement of mandibular osteotomies that are performed later on

Surgical technique

1. Condyle, capsule and meniscus are advanced onto articular eminence
2. Block of cartilage graft attached to articular fossa with wires or plates
3. MMF applied for 1 week
4. Graft calcifies so permanent advancement of condyle is obtained
5. Over a period of a few months, a new articular fossa forms anterior to the graft and the eminence appears to migrate forwards

Complications

1. Damage to external acoustic meatus
2. Graft infection
3. Facial nerve damage
4. Temporomandibular pain and dysfunction

Body procedures

Historical review

Hullihen (1849) performed an anterior subapical osteotomy to correct an anterior open bite deformity due to burns which was later modified by Kole (1965).

Blair (1907) first described a body ostectomy of the mandible.

Thoma (1943) described the Y-shaped and trapezoid ostectomies of the posterior body of mandible to correct open bites.

Indications

1. Where deformity exists in the body of the mandible, i.e. too long or short
2. Where there are missing teeth or teeth that can be sacrificed
3. Where changes in arch width are required
4. Where small corrections no more than width of a tooth is required
5. To correct reverse curve of spee, i.e. anterior open bite – more effective than ramus procedures

Complications

1. Haematoma/infection
2. Wound dehiscence
3. Airway obstruction – postop oedema
4. Sensory disturbance to lower lip
5. Delayed union
6. Non-union
7. Increased morbidity – operating time much longer than for ramus surgery

Body ostectomies/mandibuloplasty (*Fig. 4.3a* and *b*)

1. Anterior to mental foramen

To correct mandibular arch width discrepancies .

a. Step osteotomy/ostectomy
b. Midline symphyseal
c. Sowray–Haskell procedure – used to narrow mandibular arch and reduce mandible in the AP direction

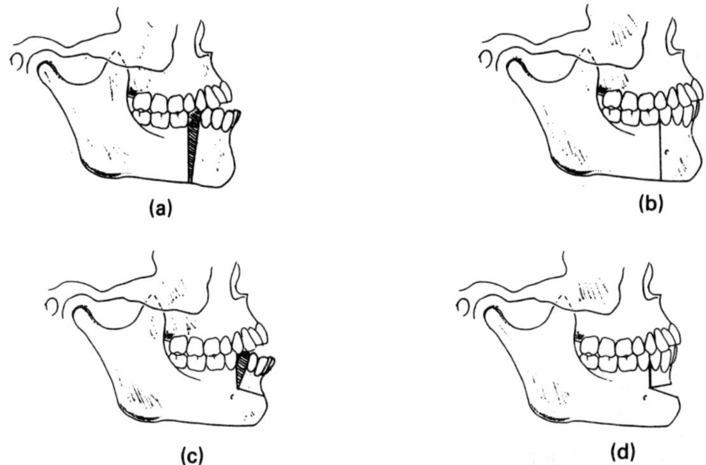

Figure 4.3 Mandibular body procedures. (a) Mandibular body ostectomy with premolar extraction. (b) Postoperative result of corrected open bite. (c) Anterior subapical procedure with premolar extraction. (d) Postoperative result. NB: gap is usually bone grafted.

2. Posterior to mental foramen

To correct reverse mandibular curve of Spee and large discrepancies in mandibular body length.

a. Y-ostectomy
b. Rectangular ostectomy
c. Trapeziod ostectomy
d. Inverted 'V' ostectomy

Note: Careful dissection of the inferior alveolar neurovascular bundle along the mandibular canal is an important and complicated part of the procedure.

3. Mandibuloplasty

Where the lower border of the mandible is trimmed to correct a mandibular asymmetry caused by bowing of the inferior border on the hyperplastic side of the mandible. Must be careful to avoid inferior alveolar neurovascular bundle which may be close to the inferior border – if encountered, it must be carefully repositioned superiorly.

Subapical osteotomies (*Fig. 4.3c* and *d*)

Few indications – cases of abnormal dentoalveolar relationship associated with minor degrees of malocclussion where orthodontics is impractical, i.e. time factor, patient preference.

Anterior subapical osteotomy (Hullihen 1849)

Indications

1. To advance or retrude lower anterior segment
2. To close anterior open bite

Technique

1. Vestibular incision
2. Identify mental nerve
3. Osteotomy cuts made 5 mm below root apices
4. Anterior dentoalveolar segment retains a lingual soft tissue pedicle which must be preserved to prevent devitalization of segment
5. Fixation of segments

Kole procedure (1965) (*Fig. 4.3c* and *d*)

1. A modification of the standard anterior segmental osteotomy to correct anterior open bite
2. Portion from lower border of mandible (chin point) is removed, trimmed and inserted into the gap produced by raising the anterior segment. *This step is of historical interest only since allogenic bone or other graft material is now used instead*

Symphyseal osteotomy

Used to narrow arch width. It is almost never used alone; it is most commonly combined with a BSSO (bilateral sagittal split osteotomy). It can also be combined with subapical anterior osteotomy.

Posterior subapical osteotomy

1. A technically difficult procedure reserved for supereruption of posterior mandibular teeth since the vascular supply is easily compromised

2. Requires isolation of the whole length of inferior alveolar nerve and retension of a soft tissue pedicle on the lingual side
3. Minimum 5 mm cut below tooth apices

Total subapical osteotomy

Limited indications

1. Increase height of mandible
2. Levelling of occlusal plane

Technique

1. Horizontal subapical cut below inferior dental canal from third molar to third molar via vestibular degloving incision
2. Sagittal split of ramus which joins vertical cut through lateral cortex
3. Mobilization and fixation as for sagittal split osteotomy

Further reading

Banks P and Ardouin DG (1980) The post-condylar graft in the treatment of disto-occlusion – a preliminary report. *Br. J. Oral Surg.* **18**, 17.

Banks P and MacKenzie L (1975) Criteria for condylotomy: a clinical appraisal of 211 cases. *Proc. R. Soc. Med.* **68**, 601.

Bell WH, Proffit WR and White PR (1980) *Surgical Correction of Dentofacial Deformities.* Vols 1 and 2. WB Saunders, Philadelphia.

Bell WH and Schendel SA (1977) Biological basis for modification of the sagittal ramus split operation. *J. Oral Surg.* **35**, 362.

Blair VP (1907) Operations on jaw bones and face. *Gynecol. Obstet.* **4**, 67.

Caldwell JB and Letterman GS (1954) Vertical osteotomy in the mandibular rami for correction of prognathism. *J. Oral Surg.* **12**, 185.

Caldwell JB, Hayward JR and Lister RL (1968) Correction of mandibular retrognathia by vertical L-osteotomy: a new technique. *J. Oral Surg.* **26**, 259.

Dalpont G (1961) Retromolar osteotomy for the correction of prognathism. *J. Oral Surg.* **19**, 42.

Epker BN, Wolford LM and Fish LC (1978) Mandibular deficiency syndrome: surgical considerations for mandibular advancement. *Oral Surg.* **45**, 349.

Epker BN and Wolford LM (1980) *Dentofacial Deformities*. CV Mosby, St Louis.

Epker BN and Fish LC (1986) *Dentofacial Deformities: Integrated Orthodontic–Surgical Correction.* CV Mosby, St Louis.

Hullihen SP (1849) Case of elongation of the under jaw and distortion of the face and neck, caused by a burn, successfully treated. *Am. J. Dent. Sci.* **9**, 157.

Hunsuck EE (1968) Modified intraoral sagittal split technique for correction of mandibular prognathism. *J. Oral Surg.* **26**, 249.

Kole B (1959) Surgical operations on the alveolar ridge to correct occlusal abnormalities. *J. Oral Surg.* **12**, 277.

Kole H (1965) In: Reischenback, Kole, Brueckel (ed): *Chirurgische Kieferorthopadie*. Barth, Leipzig.

Kostecka F (1931) Die chirurgische therapie der progenie. *Zahnartzliche Rundschau* **40**, 669.

Pichler H and Trauner R (1948) *Mund und Kieferchirurgie*. Part II, Vols 1 & 2. Wein, Urban and Schwarzenberg.

Proffit WR and White RP (1991) *Surgical–Orthodontic Treatment.* Mosby Year Book, St Louis.

Thoma KH (1943) Y-shaped osteotomy for correction of open-bite in adults. *Am. J. Orthod. and Oral Surg.* **29**, 472.

Trauner R (1954) Die retrokondylar implantation. *Deutsche Zahn. Mund. Keiferheilk.* **20**, 391.

Trauner R and Obwegeser HL (1957) The surgical correction of mandibular prognathism and retrognathia with consideration of genioplasty. *Oral Surg.* **10**, 677.

Upton LG and Sullivan SM (1990) Modified condylotomies for management of mandibular prognathism and TMJ internal derangement. *J. Clin. Orthod.* **24**, 697.

Ward TG (1961) Surgery of the mandibular joint. *Ann. R. College. Surg.* **28**, 139.

Wolford LM, Hilliard FW and Dugan DJ (1985) *Surgical Treatment Objectives: A Systematic Approach to the Prediction Tracing*. CV Mosby, St Louis.

Chapter 5

Midface surgery

Introduction

Historical review

Langenbeck (1860s) was the first to describe the maxillary osteotomy in Europe.

Cheever (1867) as reported by Moloney *et al*. 1981. A Boston surgeon performed the first LeFort I maxillary osteotomy for access to a nasopharyngeal tumour.

Cohn-Stock (1921) described the first anterior maxillary osteotomy to correct an anterior open bite.

Wassmund (1927) reported in his 1935 textbook, a LeFort I maxillary osteotomy to correct an anterior open bite. The maxilla was only partially sectioned from its bony attachments but *not* mobilized at the time of surgery. Intermaxillary elastic traction was used postoperatively to close the open bite.

Axhausen (1934). The first to advance a maxilla at the LeFort I level which was incompletely mobilized at the time of operation but postop elastics were used.

Schuchardt (1942). To prevent impairment of the vascular supply to the maxilla, a two-stage procedure was devised. The second stage involved separation of the maxilla at the pterygoid plates. Postop, weights hung from an overhead traction device were used to advance the maxilla.

Gillies and Harrison (1950) performed the first LeFort III osteotomy in 1941 which was later made routine by Tessier in the 1960s.

Converse and Shapiro (1952) advanced the maxilla by means of a transverse palatal cut at the junction of the palatine and maxillary bone.

Bell (1969–75). In his experiments on adult rhesus monkeys, established the scientific basis for the safety of LeFort I downfracture osteotomy with full mobilization under direct vision.

Obwegeser (1969) described a very high level LFI osteotomy whereby interpositional bone grafts were placed in pterygoid plate region to aid stability in large advancements. Also advocated the use of simultaneous LFI and LFIII procedures.

Kufner (1971), Converse et al. (1970), Henderson and Jackson (1973) described various approaches to the LeFort II osteotomy.

Bennett and Wolford (1985) developed the LeFort I 'STEP' osteotomy which allowed bone cuts to be made parallel to Frankfurt horizontal plane.

Types of midface osteotomies

Segmental maxillary surgery

1. Single tooth osteotomy
2. Corticotomy
3. Anterior segmental osteotomy
   a. Wassmund (1935)
   b. Wunderer (1963)
   c. Epker and Wolford (1980)
4. Posterior segmental osteotomy
   a. Schuchardt (1959)
   b. Kufner (1971)
5. Horseshoe osteotomy
   - Wolford and Epker (1975)

Total maxillary surgery

1. LeFort I osteotomy
   a. Classic downfracture (Bell 1969–75)
   b. Surgically assisted maxillary expansion (buttress release)
   c. Quadrangular (Keller and Sather 1990)
2. LeFort II osteotomy
   a. Anterior LFII osteotomy (Converse *et al*. 1970)
   b. Pyramidal LFII osteotomy (Henderson and Jackson, 1973)
   c. Quadrangular LFII osteotomy (Kufner, 1971)

3. LeFort III osteotomy

   a. Gillies (1940s)
   b. Tessier (1950s and 60s)

4. Other midface osteotomies

   a. Zygomatic osteotomies
   b. Malar–maxillary osteotomy (Obwegeser 1969) – malars attached as wings to maxilla

Segmental maxillary osteotomies

Basic principles of segmental maxillary surgery

1. Surgical repositioning of small dentoalveolar segments is possible provided maximal palatal and labiobuccal mucoperiosteal attachment is maintained
2. Design of bone and soft tissue incisions should aim for the largest possible dento-osseous segment in order to preserve the greatest amount of soft tissue pedicle
3. Inadvertent injury to cementum in the midportion of a tooth frequently heals without problem, but inadvertent apicectomy of teeth may initiate progressive pulpal atrophy and fibrous degeneration resulting in devitalization despite pulpal and osseous revascularization

Single tooth osteotomies

Limited mainly to upper anterior teeth which are dilacerated or traumatically impacted.

Incision – either high vestibular cut or two vertical incisions on either side of tooth. Flap should only be raised at the osteotomy sites and not over tooth itself.

Osteotomy – 3 mm apical to root apex and at least 2–3 mm from alveolar crest. Separated with fine osteotomes. Fixed to adjacent teeth with interdental wires for several weeks.

Corticotomy

To permit surgically assisted retraction of upper anterior teeth in class II div. I malocclusions. Via a vestibular incision first premolar to first premolar, sections of cortical bone are removed between each tooth labially and palatally. Bone is also removed 5 mm above the apices of teeth and heavy orthodontic traction is then applied for 6–12 weeks.

Posterior segmental maxillary osteotomy (*Fig. 5.1*)

A seldom used procedure first described by Schuchardt (1959) as a two-stage procedure which was later modified by Kufner (1968) as a one-stage operation. Recently reviewed by Moloney *et al.* (1984).

Indications

1. Correction of anterior (impaction) or posterior (downgraft) open bite
2. Correction of posterior crossbites (expansion)
3. Closure of existing edentulous spaces as in cleft cases (advancement)
4. Creation of space in arch for impacted canine or premolar tooth (set-back)
5. Impaction of supererupted maxillary teeth

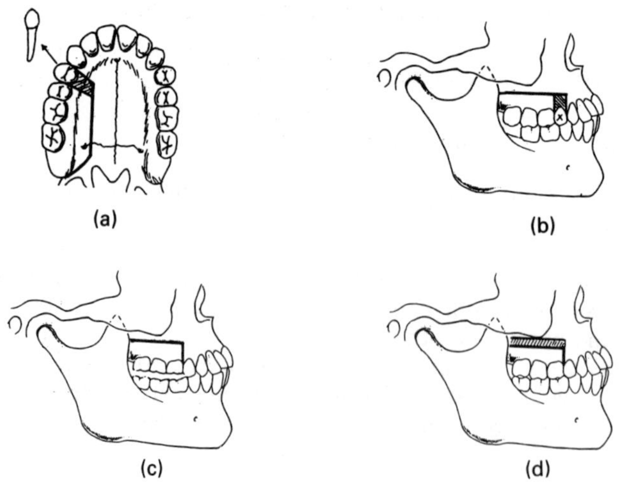

Figure 5.1 Posterior segmental maxillary osteotomy. (a) Palatal view of advancement posterior segmental maxillary osteotomy. (b) Lateral view of advancement posterior segmental maxillary osteotomy. (c) Posterior segmental maxillary osteotomy to correct posterior open bite. (d) Downgrafted posterior maxillary segment.

Technique

- Horizontal buccal incision
- Osteotomies made through mucoperiosteal tunnels in buccal plate and palate
- Fixation by archbars, MMF and occlusal wafer

Horseshoe osteotomy

Wolford and Epker 1975. Palate remains in original position as the dentoalveolar complex is repositioned superiorly by telescoping it over the hard palate.

The aim is to minimize the reduction in size of the nasal cavity, hence airway, which is produced by superior impaction of maxilla.

There are relatively few absolute indications for its use since in clinical practice there is no apparent compromise of the nasal airway even with large maxillary impactions.

In addition, it is technically difficult to position segments because of the multiple areas of bony contact.

Anterior segmental maxillary osteotomy (*Fig. 5.2*)

Where alteration of the premaxilla in the vertical plane is required as in anterior open bite or deep overbite. Three techniques are described but the downfracture technique is preferable when vertical movement is needed.

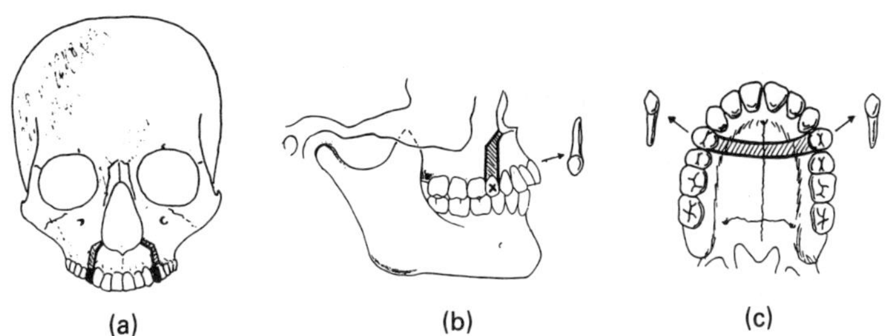

Figure 5.2 Anterior segmental maxillary osteotomy. (a) Frontal view of set-back procedure. (b) Lateral view – note the extraction of premolars. (c) Palatal view – shaded area shows ostectomy to set-back the anterior segment.

Wassmund technique (*1935*)

Incisions

- Vertical incisions in premolar region and along frenum
- Midline sagittal incision along hard palate

Osteotomy

- Bone cuts made via tunnelling approach under mucosa
- Buccal – right angled osteotomy with extraction of 1st premolars
- Sublabial – separation of nasal septum and lateral nasal wall
- Palatal – transverse cut from first premolar to first premolar by tunnelling beneath mucosa

There is normally 10–15 mm of bone between nasal floor and tooth apices.

Wunderer technique (*1963*)

Similar to Wassmund, except the palate is exposed by a transverse palatal incison with the margins away from osteotomy site.

Epker and Wolford downfracture technique (1980)

Approach is via a short vestibular incision as for LeFort I osteotomies. All bone cuts including those of the palate are performed from the labiobuccal side in a semiblind fashion making sure bur does not penetrate through intact palatal mucosa. Separation is completed by osteotome and downfractured using finger pressure.

Total maxillary osteotomies

LeFort I osteotomy (*Fig. 5.3*)

Classic LeFort I downfracture (*Fig. 5.3a*)

Bell et al. (*1969–75*) laid the biological foundations for the safety of the LeFort I downfracture osteotomy. Using 14 adult rhesus monkeys, they undertook microangiographic and histological studies of total maxillary osteotomy undergoing healing at various time intervals. They found:

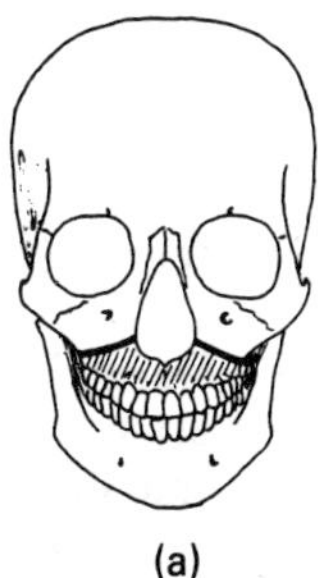

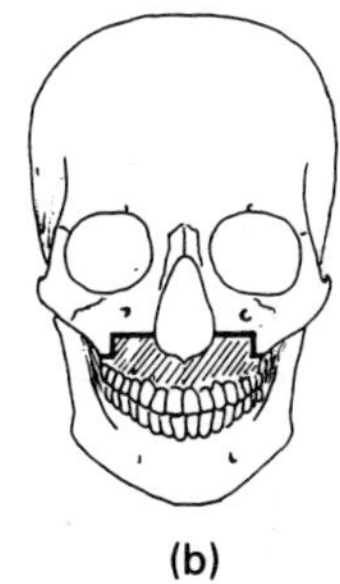

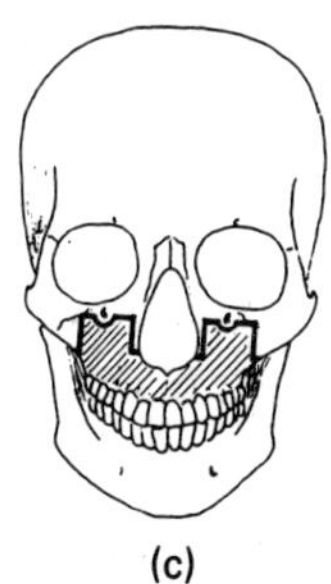

Figure 5.3 Variations of the LeFort I maxillary osteotomy. (a) Classic horizontal osteotomy. (b) Step osteotomy (Bennet and Wolford 1985). (c) Quadrangular osteotomy (Keller and Sather 1990).

1. Only transient vascular ischaemia
2. Minimal osteonecrosis
3. Early osseous union

Their results hence demonstrated:

1. As long as the maxilla is pedicled to palatal mucosa and labiobuccal gingivae and mucosa, there was adequate nutrient pedicles required for LeFort I downfracture and maxillary viability
2. Segmentalization, stretching of vascular pedicles and transection of the descending palatine vessels had *no* discernible effect on revascularization or bone healing associated with LeFort I osteotomies

Bell's work permitted technical advances in total maxillary surgery such as:

1. Allowing full mobilization of maxilla hence reducing risk of relapse
2. Permitting bone surgery under direct vision

Surgical technique

1. Vestibular incision first molar to first molar. *Previous palatal surgery may compromise palatal blood supply to segmented maxilla, whereby vertical incisions and subperiosteal tunnelling should be used instead.*

2. LeFort I level osteotomy at least 5 mm above apices of teeth.

    a. Straight line osteotomies create a ramping effect hence simple advancements would also result in decreased vertical height (*Fig. 5.4a*).
    b. Step osteotomy (Bennett and Wolford, 1985) (*Fig. 5.3b*) allowed horizontal bone cuts to be made parallel to Frankfurt horizontal, permitting horizontal maxillary movements without altering vertical dimensions hence 'ramping' effects are minimized (*Fig. 5.4b*).

        i. Anterior cut 4–5 mm above canine apices
        ii. Vertical cut – zygomatic buttress region (*excellent site for bone grafts*)
        iii. Posterior cuts 4–5 mm above molar apices

3. Osteotomy of lateral nasal wall and nasal septum
4. Separation of pterygomaxillary junction

    - First advocated by Axhausen in 1934 by use of the curved osteotome
    - The correct use of curved osteotome and review of regional anatomy was described by Turvey and Fonseca (1980)
    - Precious *et al*. (1991) have described pterygomaxillary separation without osteotome
    - Complications of unfavourable dysjunction in this region include:

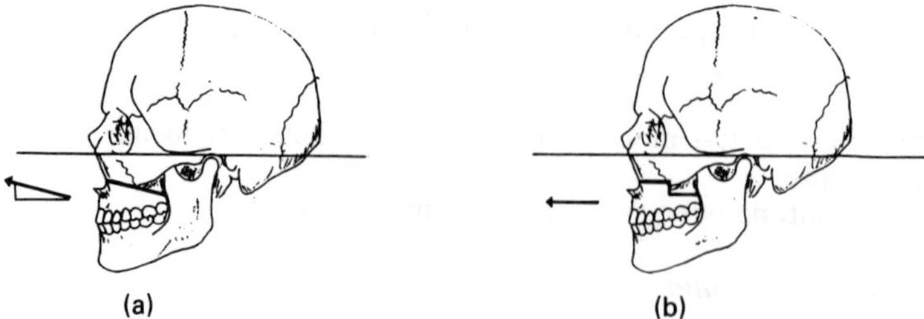

Figure 5.4 Comparative geometry of maxillary advancement. (a) Classic 'horizontal' osteotomy results in ramping effect or changes in vertical position of maxilla with horizontal movements at the LeFort I level. (b) Step osteotomy cuts are made parallel to Frankfurt horizontal ensuring minimal change in vertical position with horizontal movements of the maxilla.

a. Excessive bleeding
b. Cranial nerve injury
c. Carotid artery injury

5. Downfracture of maxilla

- Rowe's dissimpaction forceps sometimes used
- Hypotensive anaesthesia is desirable to minimize blood loss

6. Complete mobilization and trimming of maxilla

- Maxilla must be able to sit passively in new position
- The pyramidal strut of bone surrounding the descending palatine arteries must be removed to allow posterior impaction (Johnson and Arnett 1991)
- Lateral nasal walls and septum must all be carefully trimmed back

7. Fixation

- For advancements > 5 mm and downgrafts, stability and healing is greatly facilitated by interpositional bone grafts especially in the buttress region (direct vision) and pterygomaxillary junction (blindly)

Quadrangular LeFort I osteotomy (*Fig. 5.3c*)

As first reported by Keller and Sather (1990), who reviewed 54 patients. This is similar to the quadrangular LFII osteotomy as described below, with the exception that the inferior orbital rims are not mobilized.

Indications. Similar to that of quadrangular LFII (i.e. receded inferior orbital margins, zygomas and maxilla, but with normal nasal projection) except it is also possible to use where there is significant maxillary midline shifts (> 2 mm) and maxillary vertical (> 5 mm) and transverse discrepancies which cannot be normally corrected with the LFII procedure. More versatile than quadrangular LFII osteotomy.

Technical aspects. It is basically a high LFI osteotomy that incorporates almost all anterolateral aspects of maxilla below infraorbital nerve and parts of body of malar. Miniplate fixation in the periorbital areas is difficult because of poor access through intraoral approach and insufficient bone in area although interpositional grafts have aided stability and minimized MMF.

Complications. In addition to those seen in classic LFI procedures, the following may also occur:

1. Irregular infraorbital contour – LFII quadrangular osteotomies provide better aesthetics in this area
2. Nasolacrimal duct dysfunction

LeFort II osteotomy (*Fig. 5.5*)

Steinhauser (1980) provided an excellent review of LFII osteotomies and classified them into three types.

Anterior LF2 osteotomy (*Fig. 5.5a*)

The problem of nasomaxillary hypoplasia has been addressed by Converse *et al.* (1970) who discussed its aetiology at length and proposed a pyramidal nasoorbital maxillary osteotomy that combined an intraoral premaxillary osteotomy, but did not include posterior maxilla or infraorbital rims.

Pyramidal LFII osteotomy (*Fig. 5.5b*)

Henderson and Jackson (1973) wrote a paper describing an osteotomy approximating the LeFort II fracture pattern and discussed its indications, viz nasomaxillary hypoplasia

1. Including dentoalveolar segment

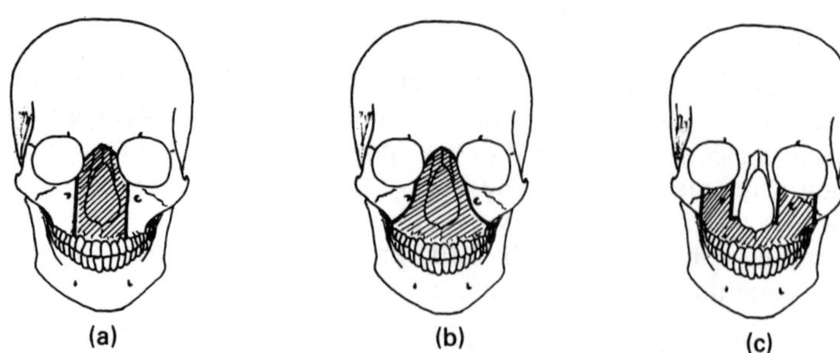

Figure 5.5 Variations of the LeFort II midface osteotomy. (a) Anterior osteotomy (Converse *et al*. 1970). (b) Pyramidal osteotomy (Henderson and Jackson 1973). (c) Quadrangular osteotomy (Keller and Sather 1987 and others).

2. Excluding dentoalveolar segment
3. Involving cleft palate cases
4. Involving other facial dysharmonies

Technique. Osteotomy cuts followed closely LeFort II fracture pattern via coronal incision and intraoral approach with interpositional bone grafts and tracheostomy being performed in all seven cases.

Quadrangular LF2 osteotomy (Fig. 5.5c)

First described by Kufner (1971) and subsequently modified by Souyris *et al*. (1973), Champy (1980) and Steinhauser (1980) who coined the term 'quadrangular'.

Indications. This modified LFII osteotomy is used for patients with significant maxillary deficiency that extends to the infraorbital rims and zygomas but who have normal nasal projection.

Keller and Sather (1987) recently described a wholly intraoral approach to the quadrangular LFII osteotomy in seven patients. Fixation was accomplished by transosseous wires and interpositional bone grafts. The technique involves osteotomies that incorporate the inferior orbital margin, infraorbital nerve and body of zygoma which are attached to the maxilla as one piece and advanced or impacted, provided there is no more than 2 mm midline shift descrepancy of the maxilla, as well as <5 mm vertical and transverse discrepancies.

LeFort III osteotomies (see Chapter 11)

The first total midface osteotomy at LeFort III level was reported by Gillies and Harrison in 1950. However, extensive pioneering work by Tessier in the 1960s established the feasibility of routinely performing the LFIII osteotomy to correct severe midfacial congenital deformities as commonly found in the craniofacial dysostoses such as Aperts, Crouzon and Pfieffer syndromes.

Technical aspects

In syndrome patients the LFIII osteotomy is usually performed at an early age (e.g. 7 years) with a LFI osteotomy undertaken later on at the cessation of growth.

Relapse

In non-growing patients, LFIII osteotomies appear to be quite stable procedures. When undertaken in young growing children, relapse that does occur is related to continued mandibular growth rather than midface relapse (Kaban *et al*. 1986). Interpositional bone grafts play an important role in stability.

Further reading

Axhausen G (1934) Zur Behandlung veralteter disloziert geheitter Oberkieferbruche. *Dtsch. Zahn. Mund. Kieferheilk.* **1**, 334.

Bachmayer D, Ross B and Munro I (1986) Maxillary growth following LeFort III advancement surgery in Crouzon, Apert and Pfeiffer syndromes. *Am. J. Orthod.* **90**, 420.

Bell WH (1969) Revascularization and bone healing after anterior maxillary osteotomy: a study using rhesus monkeys. *J. Oral Surg.* **27**, 249.

Bell WH (1973) Biological basis for maxillary osteotomies. *Am. J. Phys. Anthropol.* **38**, 279.

Bell WH, Fonseca RJ, Kennedy JW *et al*. (1975) Bone healing and revascularization after total maxillary osteotomy. *J. Oral Surg.* **33**, 253.

Bennett MA and Wolford LM (1985) The maxillary step osteotomy and Steinmann pin stabilization. *J. Oral Maxillofac. Surg.* **43**, 307.

Champy M (1980) Surgical treatment of midface deformities. *Head Neck Surg.* **2**, 451.

Cohn-Stock G (1921) Die chirurgische Immediatre-gulierung der Kiefer, speziell die chirurgische. *Behuandlung der Prognathie, Vjschr Zahnheilk Berlin* **37**, 320.

Converse JM and Shapiro HH (1952) Treatment of developmental malformations of the jaws. *Plast. Reconstr. Surg.* **10**, 316.

Drommer RB (1986) The history of the LeFort I osteotomy. *J. Maxillofac. Surg.* **14**, 119.

Epker BN and Wolford LM (1975) Middle third face osteotomies: their use in the correction of acquired and developmental craniofacial deformities. *J. Oral Surg.* **33**, 491.

Epker BN and Fish LC (1986) *Dentofacial Deformities: Integrated Orthodontic-Surgical correction.* CV Mosby, St Louis.

Epker BN and Schendel SA (1980) Total maxillary surgery. *Int. J. Oral Surg.* **9**, 1.

Epker BN and Wolford LM (1980) *Dentofacial Deformities*. CV Mosby, St Louis.

Fish LC and Epker BN (1987) Dentofacial deformities related to midface deficiencies. *J. Clin. Orthod.* **21**, 654.

Gillies H and Harrison SH (1950) Operative correction by osteotomy of recessed malar-maxillary complex in a case of oxycephaly. *Br. J. Plast. Surg.* **3**, 123.

Henderson D and Jackson IT (1973) Nasomaxillary hypoplasia – the LeFort II osteotomy. *Br. J. Oral Surg.* **11**, 77.

Johnson LM and Arnett GW (1991) Pyramidal osseous release around the descending palatine artery: a surgical technique. *J. Oral Maxillofac. Surg.* **49**, 1356.

Kaban LB, Conover M and Mulliken JB (1986) Midface position after LeFort III advancement: a long term follow-up study. *Cleft Palate J. Suppl.* **23**, 75.

Keller EE and Sather AH (1987) Intraoral quadrangular LeFort II osteotomy. *J. Oral Maxillofac. Surg.* **45**, 223.

Keller EE and Sather AH (1990) Quadrangular LeFort I osteotomy: Surgical technique and review of 51 patients. *J. Oral Maxillofac. Surg.* **48**, 2.

Kraut RA (1984) Surgically assisted rapid maxillary expansion by opening the midpalatal suture. *J. Oral Maxillofac. Surg.* **42**, 651.

Kufner J (1971) Four years experience with major maxillary osteotomy for retrusion. *Oral Surg.* **29**, 549.

Langenbeck BV (1859) Beitrage zur osteoplastik – Die osteoplastische resektion des oberkiefers. In: Goshen A (ed): *Deutsche Klinik.* Reimer, Berlin.

Moloney F, Stoelinger PJW and Tideman H (1984) The posterior segmental maxillary osteotomy: recent applications. *J. Oral Maxillofac. Surg.* **42**, 771.

Moloney F and Worthington P (1981) The origin of the LeFort I maxillary osteotomy. Cheever's operation. *J. Oral Surg.* **39**, 731.

Obwegeser HL (1969) Surgical correction of small or retrodisplaced maxillae. *Plast. Reconstr. Surg.* **43**, 351.

Precious D, Morrison A and Ricard D (1991) Pterygomaxillary separation without the use of an osteotome. *J. Oral Maxillofac. Surg.* **49**, 98.

Proffit WR and White RP (1991) *Surgical–Orthodontic Treatment*. Mosby Year Book, St Louis.

Schuchardt K (1942) Ein Beitrag zur chirurgischen Kieferorthopadie unter Berucksichtigung. *Dtsch Zahn Mund Kieferhk* **9**, 73.

Schuchardt K (1959) Experiences with the surgical treatment of deformities of the jaws: prognathia, micrognathia and open bite. In: Wallace AC (ed): *Second Congress of International Society of Plastic Surgeons*, London, Livingstone.

Steinhauser EW (1980) Variations of LeFort II osteotomies for correction of midface deformities. *J. Maxillofac. Surg.* **8**, 258.

Tessier P (1971) Total osteotomy of the middle third of the face for faciostenosis or for sequelae of Le Fort III fractures. *Plast. Reconstr. Surg.* **48**, 533.

Turvey TA and Fonseca RJ (1980) The anatomy of the internal maxillary artery in the pterygopalatine fossa: its relationship to maxillary surgery. *J. Oral Surg.* **38**, 92.

Wassmund J (1935) *Lehrbuch der Praktischen Chirugie de Mundes und der Kiefer.* Vol 1. Meusser, Leipzig.

Wolford LM, Hilliard FW and Dugan DJ (1985) *Surgical Treatment Objectives: A Systematic Approach to the Prediction Tracing.* CV Mosby, St Louis.

Wunderer S (1963) Erfahrungen mit der operativen Behandlung hochgradiger Prognathien. *Dtsch Zahn Mund Kieferheilk* **39**, 451.

Chapter 6

Orthognathic procedures

Introduction

With the establishment of the scientific basis for the various orthognathic surgical techniques, it has become possible to apply these procedures to the treatment of the numerous dentofacial deformities. The most commonly used orthognathic techniques are the LeFort I downfracture for the maxilla and the ramus osteotomy techniques for the mandible, in particular the sagittal split and the vertical subsigmoid osteotomies. This chapter will deal with the application of these most commonly used orthognathic surgical techniques for the management of the more common dentofacial deformities as outlined in Chapter 1.

Terminology of common orthognathic procedures

The most commonly performed orthognathic procedures involve the movement of the jaws in any one or combination of the following directions relative to the cranial base:

1. Maxillary surgery – permits the movement of the tooth-bearing segments of the maxilla in the following directions:

a. Vertical

i. Superior repositioning (*impaction*)
ii. Inferior repositioning (*downgraft*)

b. Horizontal

i. Anteroposterior (*advancement*)
ii. Transverse (*expansion*)

2. Mandibular surgery – the mandible may be moved in the following directions:

a. Horizontal (anteroposterior)

   i. Advancement
   ii. Set-back

b. Vertical (autorotation) – this is often the result of vertical changes in the maxilla that gives rise to the following vertical movements of the mandible without necessarily undertaking surgery in the mandible itself:

   i. Clockwise – results in decreased chin projection
   ii. Counter-clockwise – results in greater chin projection

Maxillary surgery (LeFort I downfracture procedures)

Maxillary impaction (superior repositioning) (*Fig. 6.1*)

Indications

Vertical maxillary excess (VME) with:

- Open bite
- No open bite

Aesthetics

Deformity mainly in vertical facial balance (long face – dolicofacial)

1. Relatively long lower third of face

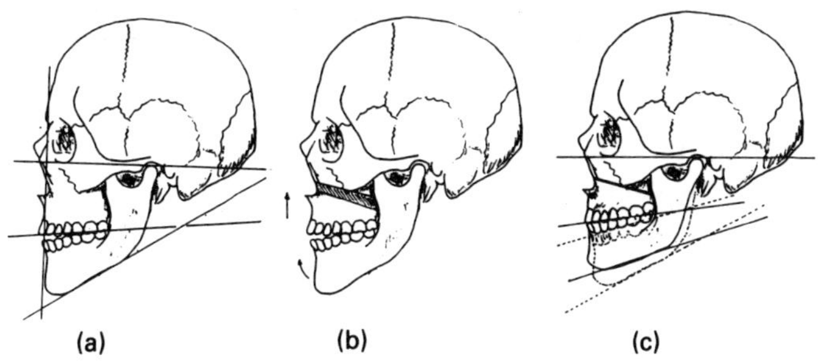

Figure 6.1 Dolicofacial – vertical maxillary excess with open bite.
(a) Cephalometric features – high mandibular plane angle. (b) LeFort I maxillary impaction. (c) Surgical result – mandibular autorotation results in corrected open bite, decreased occlusal plane and mandibular plane angles.

2. Lip incompetence with excessive exposure of teeth and gingivae
3. With open bite – excessive eversion and exposure of lower lip at rest
4. No open bite – excessive tooth display with narrow alar base of nose
5. Profile

    a. Nasal prominence
    b. Marked interlabial distance
    c. Recessive chin especially with open bite cases

Occlusion

1. Class II malocclusion
2. V-shaped upper arches
3. Open bite – maxillary crowding with posterior crossbites

Cephalometric features (*Fig. 6.1a*)

1. Large lower facial height resulting from long posterior facial height
2. Relative mandibular retrognathia with high mandibular plane angle

Treatment planning (*Fig. 6.1b*)

Ideal upper incisal exposure is 2–3 mm (Burstone 1967) stomion to incisal tip. With maxillary impaction, upper lip moves 1 mm (20%) for every 5 mm of superior repositioning of front teeth. With maxillary impactions, mandible rotates counterclockwise which:

1. Shortens the lower face
2. Makes the chin more prominent

Surgical procedure

1. VME without open bite. One piece maxillary osteotomy with careful trimming of bony interferences which may prevent maxilla from seating passively in superior position, e.g. pyramidal bony release around descending palatine artery.

2. *VME with open bite (see below)* (*Fig. 6.1b* and *c*). Differential impaction of maxilla, which may also require bimaxillary surgery. Segmental maxillary surgery may be required to correct transverse maxillary problem. Greater than 5 mm impaction may require horseshoe osteotomy to minimize decrease in nasal airway. However, studies have demonstrated that this is unnecessary.

Maxillary downgraft (inferior repositioning) (*Fig. 6.2*)

Indications

1. Vertical maxillary deficiency (short face – brachyfacial)
2. Maxillary atrophy due to prolonged edentulous state

Aesthetics

1. Poor incisal display even on smiling with eversion of lower lip
2. Dimunitive anterior dentoalveolar height in both jaws

Occlusal features

1. Usually class I but sometimes class II malocclusion with dental crowding
2. Deep anterior overbite
3. Wide maxilla

Cephalometric features (*Fig. 6.2a*)

1. Negative incisal display with normal AP postion of maxilla

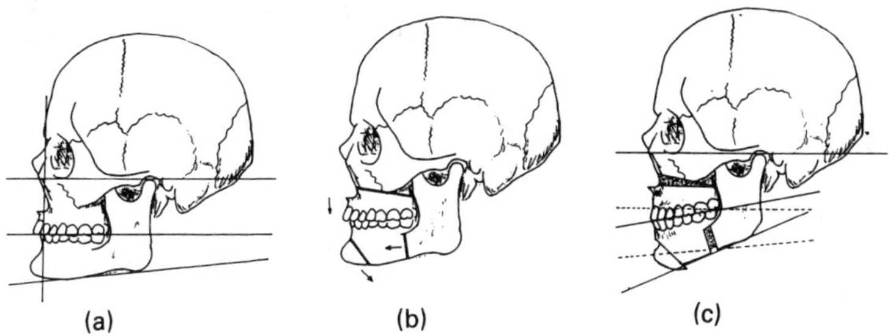

Figure 6.2 Brachyfacial – vertical maxillary deficiency. (a) Cephalometric features – low occlusal and mandibular plane angles with class II malocclusion. (b) Bimaxillary surgery and genioplasty. (c) Maxillary downgraft, mandibular advancement and set-back genioplasty.

2. Square jaw – with low almost parallel mandibular and occlusal plane angles
3. Prominent pogonion and labiomental fold

Surgical procedure (*Fig. 6.2b* and *c*)

1. Interpositional bone grafting is essential for all downgrafting procedures because of its inherently high relapse rate. Aim for overcorrection >3 mm incisal display
2. Maxillary downgrafting increases lower facial height and rotates chin downwards and backwards as occlusal and mandibular planes are increased
3. Downgrafting requires slight posterior positioning of maxilla to fit the occlusion in cases where mandibular surgery is not planned

Maxillary advancement (*Fig. 6.3*)

Indication

AP maxillary deficiency (maxillary hypoplasia)

- Non-cleft palate
- Cleft palate (see Chapter 10)

Aesthetics

1. Increased nasolabial angle
2. If nasal bridge cannot be seen in profile because the eye (globe) protrudes beyond it, it most likely needs an advancement at a higher level osteotomy

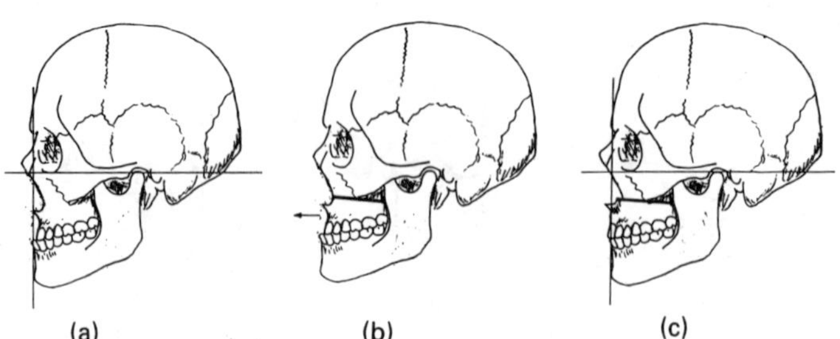

Figure 6.3 Maxillary AP deficiency (hypoplasia). (a) Class III skeletal base malocclusion. (b) Maxillary advancement. (c) Surgical result – no changes in vertical height.

3. Inadequate upper incisal display
4. Prominent everted lower lip indicative of mandibular prognathism or maxillary hypoplasia
5. Nasal balance – important preoperative measures include nasal tip, alar base width, nasolabial folds

Occlusion

1. Class III malocclusion
2. Severe dental crowding in maxilla
3. Constricted maxillary arch with posterior crossbites

Cephalometric features (*Fig. 6.3a*)

- Maxillary hypoplasia with decreased SNA angle (< 75°)
- Wide nasolabial angle

Velopharyngeal function

Of particular concern in cleft patients with short palates since maxillary advancement may well accentuate velopharyngeal incompetence (VPI). If there is a strong risk of postoperative VPI then bimaxillary surgery should be considered to minimize advancement in maxilla required for aesthetics and occlusion with onlay bone grafting in maxilla for aesthetics.

Surgical procedures (*Fig. 6.3b* and *c*)

Indications for bone grafts:

1. Maxillary advancements > 5 mm
2. Difficult cleft cases

Purpose of bone grafts (see Chapter 8):

1. To accelerate bone healing between segments
2. To serve as physical stop for increased stability and to minimize relapse
3. As onlay grafts in cases requiring > 10 mm advancement

Maxilla must be completely mobilized until it can be passively placed in desired anterior position.

Cleft patients (see Chapter 10)

1. Simultaneous expansion and grafting of alveolar clefts are readily achieved with properly designed soft tissue flaps
2. In complete cleft cases, the greater and lesser segments of maxilla are mobilized independently, otherwise must graft at least 6–12 months beforehand if single piece maxillary osteotomy is required
3. Mobilization of maxilla is difficult because of:

   a. Perpendicular plate of palatine bone
   b. Scar tissue between palate and nasal septum secondary to previous palatal surgery

Maxillary expansion

See 'crossbites' below.

Indications and clinical features

1. Transverse maxillary deficiency (bilateral/unilateral) either isolated or with class III malocclusion
2. Narrow maxilla with dental crowding
3. Few facial or cephalometric features

Treatment planning

Children. Successfully treated with orthopaedic rapid maxillary expansion.

Adults

1. Less than 5 mm transverse deficiency, orthopaedic expansion of maxilla is suffice
2. Greater than 5 mm transverse deficiency or buccally inclined posterior teeth, a combined surgical/orthodontic expansion technique is used

Combined surgical – orthodontic expansion

1. Segmental posterior alveolar osteotomy used for unilateral deficiencies
2. Lefort I downfracture with midline palatal split or horseshoe osteotomy

3. Surgically assisted rapid maxillary expansion – LeFort I osteotomy without the downfracture, and intraoperative activation of orthopaedic expansion device (see 'crossbites')

Mandibular surgery (ramus osteotomy procedures)

Mandibular deficiency

Deficiency in AP direction (*Fig. 6.4*)

- Retruded chin and lower jaw
- Crowding in lower anterior arch with overangulated incisors and accentuated curve of Spee
- Corrected by mandibular advancement with ramus osteotomies, e.g. sagittal split

Deficiency in vertical dimension

- Lower anterior dental height < 40 mm
- Sometimes mandible appears clinically short where in fact it is because of a deep overbite
- Best corrected by vertical lengthening of chin by interpositional graft and augmentation
- Deficient ramus height may be best treated with inverted 'L' osteotomy and interpositional bone graft

Deficiency in transverse dimension

- Corrected by body, symphyseal osteotomies/ostectomies or by subapical osteotomies to allow expansion of the arch

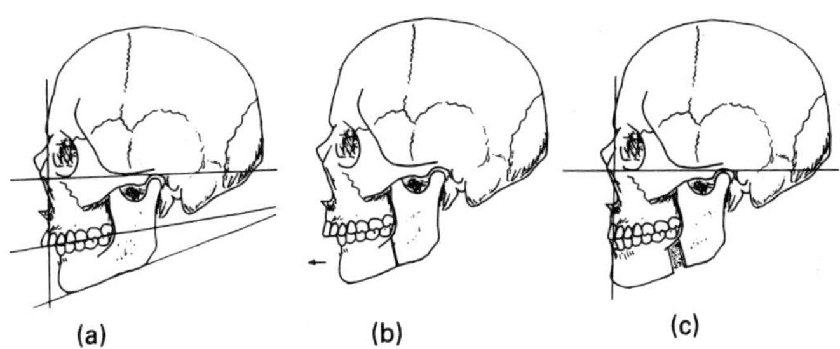

Figure 6.4 Mandibular horizontal (AP) deficiency. (a) Class II skeletal base malocclusion. (b) Sagittal split osteotomy. (c) Surgical result with mandibular advancement.

Mandibular excess

Excessive AP direction (*Fig. 6.5*)

- Mandibular prognathism with lingually inclined lower incisors
- Class III malocclusion with anterior and bilateral posterior crossbites
- Presurgical orthodontics often worsens the appearance as teeth are uprighted over basal bone prior to surgery
- Usually treated with mandibular set-back achieved via ramus osteotomies such as the sagittal split or vertical subsigmoid osteotomies

Excess vertical dimension

- Increased lower anterior dental height
- Reduction genioplasty required

Excess in transverse dimension

- Mandibular dental arch too wide in comparison to a normal maxillary arch
- Arch width can be reduced by body and symphyseal ostectomies

Double jaw surgery (*Fig. 6.2*)

Simultaneous two jaw surgery is indicated for patients with a combination of deformities affecting both jaws, so when both

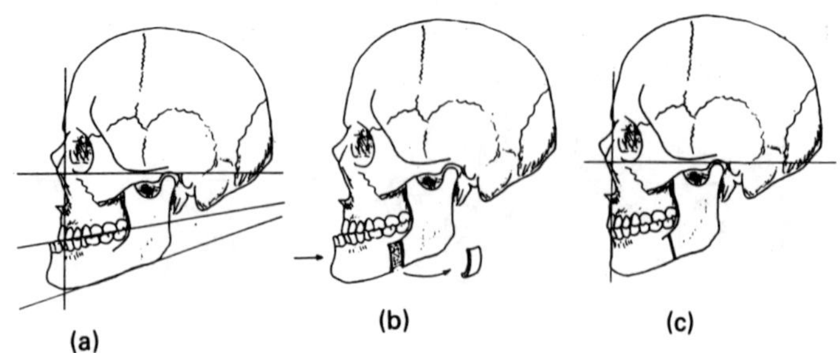

Figure 6.5 Mandibular horizontal (AP) excess. (a) Class III skeletal base malocclusion. (b) Sagittal split osteotomy with buccal plate osteotomy. (c) Surgical result with mandibular set-back.

jaws are surgically separated from the cranial base, they can then be appropriately repositioned in all three planes of space.

Double jaw surgery is usually required for:

1. Facial asymmetries
2. Combined AP problems, vertical deformities and/or transverse discrepancies

Double jaw surgery permits alterations in the occlusal plane angle which is important in balancing the chin, lips and nose

Apertognathia (*Fig. 6.1*)

Open bite – where teeth in opposing jaws fail to contact.

Aetiology

1. Anterior open bite

    a. Tongue thrust
    b. Thumb sucking
    c. Deficient eruption of anterior teeth/excessive eruption of posterior teeth
    d. Skeletal base growth discrepancy, i.e. excessive posterior facial height; severe mandibular retrognathia; short ramus height, long face syndrome
    e. Condylar resorption – idiopathic, avascular necrosis

2. Posterior open bite

    a. Deficient eruption of posterior teeth
    b. Facial asymmetry which develops after growth is completed, e.g. condylar hyperplasia (see Chapter 7)

Classification of open bites

1. Dentoalveolar
2. Skeletal base
3. Combination of both

Management

Management depends on the cause of the open bite.

1. Discourage adverse habits such as thumb or finger sucking with a variety of oral appliances which will sometimes lead to spontaneous resolution of the open bite
2. Surgical tongue reduction – tongue thrust during swallowing will create forces large enough to result in open bite. Must assess the tongue size, morphology and function in terms of:

a. True macroglossia – excessively large tongue
b. Relative macroglossia – normal size tongue confined within a restricted oral space of relatively small dental arches
c. Functional macroglossia – excessive tongue activity

The role of surgical reduction of the tongue as an adjunctive measure to the orthognathic/orthodontic management of anterior open bite is controversial.

3. Segmental orthognathic surgery – especially useful in cases of infra- or supraeruption of teeth whereby the dentoalveolar segment can be surgically repositioned anywhere in the vertical plane to close the open bite, either:

a. Directly – anterior subapical mandibular osteotomy with superior positioning to close an anterior open bite, or
b. Indirectly – posterior maxillary osteotomy with impaction which will bring the anterior segments together and close the anterior open bite

4. Total orthognathic surgery – to surgically correct the problem of open bite caused by a skeletal base discrepancy

a. Mandibular body osteotomies/ostectomies – especially useful in the correction of a reverse curve of Spee mandibular occlusal table
b. Mandibular ramus osteotomies – usually involve a counter-clockwise rotation to close the open bite which is often quite an unstable procedure with significant potential for relapse. Mainly used in cases of mandibular retrognathia where maxillary surgery is also planned
c. LeFort I maxillary osteotomy (*Fig. 6.1b* and *c*) – differential impaction of the whole maxilla yields quite a stable result and directly addresses the problem of increased posterior facial height. Probably the most favoured treatment option

Crossbites

Crossbite is where there is a reverse buccal overjet relationship of teeth in opposing jaws.

Clinical presentation

1. May occur unilaterally or bilaterally
2. Can occur anteriorly or posteriorly
3. Commonly related to a hypoplastic maxilla in a class III skeletal base malocclusion
4. Also found in cases of lower facial asymmetry (see Chapter 7).

Underlying cause

Crossbites are most frequently related to a transverse deficiency of the palatal vault or maxillary alveolar arch.

Treatment of crossbite

1. *Orthodontics* – by tipping or torquing the teeth buccally. May be unstable in cases where transverse discrepancy is > 5 mm.
2. *Skeletal* – by increasing the width of the palate via

    a. Palatal expansion devices – during growth phase
    b. Surgically assisted rapid maxillary expansion – using a combination of surgical relief of maxillary bony abutments and the use of palatal expansion devices to rapidly open up the midpalatine suture in the space of a few weeks
    c. Segmental maxillary surgery – whereby a midpalatal osteotomy is made at the time of the LeFort I maxillary downfracture to immediately expand the palate to the desired dimension in one step
    d. Segmental posterior maxillary osteotomy may be used for unilateral deficiencies or crossbites

Further reading

Egyedi P and Obwegeser H (1964) Zur operativen Zungenverk-Leineiung. *Dtsch Zahn Mund Kieferheilk* **41**, 16.

Ellis E (1985) The nature of vertical maxillary deformities: implications for surgical intervention. *J. Oral Maxillofac. Surg.* **43**, 756.

Epker BN and Fish LC (1986) *Dentofacial Deformities: Integrated Orthodontic-Surgical Correction.* CV Mosby, St Louis.

Epker BN and Schendel SA (1980) Total maxillary surgery. *Int. J. Oral Surg.* **9**, 1.
Epker BN and Wolford LM (1980) *Dentofacial Deformities*. CV Mosby, St Louis.
Fish LC, Wolford LM and Epker BN (1978) Surgical-orthodontic correction of vertical maxillary excess. *Am. J. Orthod.* **73**, 241.
Moloney F, West RA and McNeill W (1982) Surgical correction of vertical maxillary excess: a re-evaluation. *J. Maxillofac. Surg.* **10**, 84.
Opdebeeck H and Bell WH (1978). The short face syndrome. *Am. J. Orthod.* **73**, 499.
Profitt WR and White RP (eds) (1991) Crossbite and open-bite problems. In: *Surgical–Orthodontic Treatment*. Ch 16, p. 550. Mosby–Year Book, Missouri.
Speidel TM, Isaacson RJ and Worms FW (1972). Tongue thrust therapy and anterior dental open bite. *Am. J. Orthod.* **62**, 287.
Stella J, Streater M and Epker B (1989) Predictability of upper lip soft tissue changes with maxillary advancement. *Oral Maxillofac. Surg.* **47**, 697.
Trouten JC, Enlow DH, Rabine M *et al*. (1983) Morphological factors in open bite and deep bite. *Angle Orthod*. **53**, 192.
Turvey TA (1982) Simultaneous mobilization of the maxilla and mandible: surgical technique and results. *J. Oral Maxillofac. Surg.* **40**, 96.
Turvey TA (1985) Maxillary expansion: a surgical technique based on surgical–orthodontic treatment objectives and anatomic considerations. *J. Maxillofac. Surg.* **13**, 51.
Will LA (1990) Mandibular advancement using the bilateral sagittal osteotomy: past, present and future. *Oral Maxillofac. Surg. Clin. North Am.* **2**, 717.
Wolford LM and Hilliard FW (1981) The surgical–orthodontic correction of vertical dentofacial deformities. *J. Oral Surg.* **39**, 883.
Wolford LM, Hilliard FW and Dugan DJ (1985) *Surgical Treatment Objectives: A Systematic Approach to the Prediction Tracing*. CV Mosby, St Louis.

Chapter 7

Facial asymmetry

Introduction

Mechanism of lower facial asymmetry

Usually related to unbalanced aberrant growth of one side of the face, often the condylar process of the mandible, but sometimes the ramus and body may be involved.

Malocclusion may or may not be present depending on any compensatory growth in the maxilla which may have occurred. Alteration in the maxillary cant will only arise if problem emerges during normal period of facial growth, whereby compensatory growth of the maxilla will occur in relation to the aberrant mandibular growth pattern.

Clinically appears as a chin and mandibular midline shift (lower facial asymmetry).

Causes of facial asymmetry

1. Aberrant condylar growth
   a. Condylar hyperplasia
   b. Condylar hypoplasia
   c. Condylar aplasia
2. Aberrant mandibular growth
   a. Hemimandibular elongation
   b. Hemimandibular hypertrophy/hyperplasia
3. Hemifacial atrophy (Parry–Romberg syndrome)
4. Hemifacial microsomia (Goldenhar syndrome)
5. Hemifacial hypertrophy
6. Traumatic deformities (see Chapter 10)
   a. Condylar fractures
   b. Mandibular fractures (particularly of ascending ramus)

7. Neoplastic and other diseases of the facial skeleton

   a. Neurofibromatosis (von Recklinghausen's disease)
   b. Bone neoplasms, e.g. osteoma, osteosarcoma, osteochondroma (of condyle)
   c. Fibrous dysplasia
   d. Odontogenic tumours
   e. Large cystic lesions of bone, e.g. odontogenic keratocyst
   f. Temporomandibular joint ankylosis (unilateral – arising during growth)

Note: *In this section, facial asymmetry caused by growth aberration rather than disease will be presented, since orthognathic surgery does not address the disease process but only the growth anomaly.*

Clinical evaluation

1. Background history

a. When the facial asymmetry was first noticed

   i. Congenital – present at birth
   ii. Developmental – emerged sometime later

b. Progress

   i. Getting worse with time
   ii. Ceased – how long ago?

c. Any history of trauma, infection (i.e. middle ear) or surgery to the face and jaws?
d. Any close relatives such as grandparents, parents or siblings similarly affected (family pictures)?

2. Clinical examination (*Figs. 7.1* and *7.2a*)

Must remember that all normal individuals have a certain degree of facial asymmetry. Assess mainly frontal view and start from the top looking for obvious differences between left and right sides.

a. Cranial vault – e.g. plagiocephaly
b. Forehead – unilateral flattening or excess

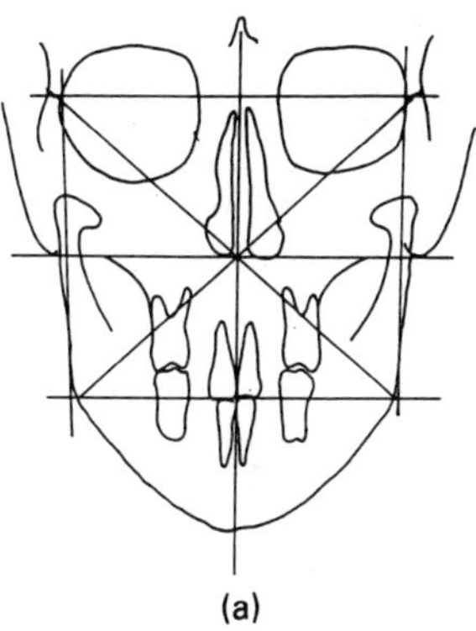

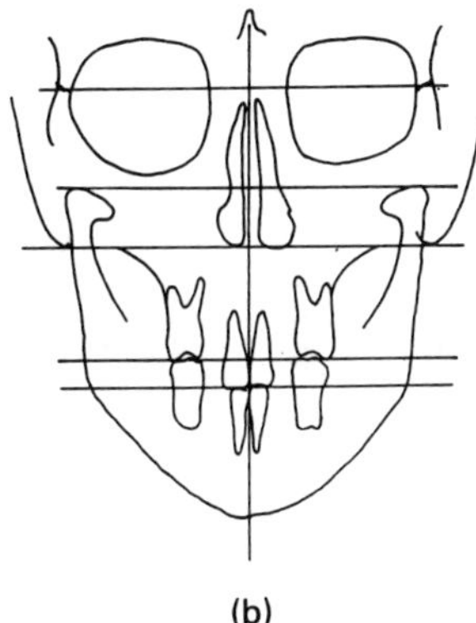

Figure 7.1 Posteroanterior (PA) cephalometric planes demonstrating a symmetrical facial skeleton. (a) Convergence of lines to anterior nasal spine. (b) Horizontal planes should be close to perpendicular with respect to vertical midline.

c. Eyes – intercanthal and interpupillary levels
d. Malar prominences
e. Nose – level of alar bases
f. Lips – level of comissures
g. Chin point – deviation from midline
h. Dental midlines
i. Maxillary occlusal cant

3. *Investigations*

a. Serial photographs – over a period of time to establish whether asymmetry is progressive or static
b. Radiographs

    i. Serial
    ii. Diagnostic (*Fig. 7.2*) – using cephalometric analysis on PA and lateral cephalograms as well as TMJ films to determine the focal cause of the asymmetry, i.e. hyperplastic condyle,

c. Radioisotopic bone scans – to determine sites of active bone growth
d. Three dimensional CT scan reconstructions
e. Biopsy – where a disease process is suspected, rather than simply just aberrant growth

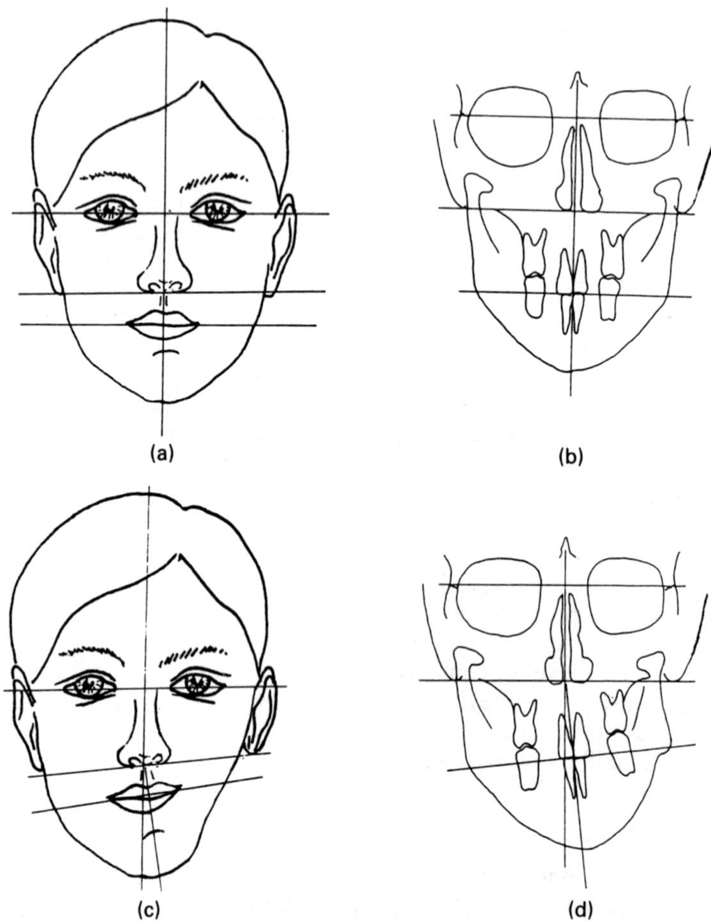

Figure 7.2 Comparison of symmetrical ((a) and (b)) and asymmetrical ((c) and (d)) facial and cephalometric features. Note the deviation of the vertical midline and accentuated angulation of the bigonion (Go–Go) plane (d) in relation to cranial base.

Principles of treatment planning

1. Must determine which side and site the abnormal growth is and where the compensatory growth has occurred
2. All disease processes must be eliminated prior to undertaking any corrective surgery
3. Often the underlying skeletal abnormalities must be first corrected prior to any soft tissue procedures. *NB: it may be*

sometimes necessary to undertake tissue expansion in deficient regions prior to the bony surgery

4. The surgery must not only aim to correct the site of aberrant growth, but also to eliminate any compensatory growth which may have occurred
5. In growing children, functional appliance therapy is of immense value particularly in the mild lower facial asymmetry cases
6. In the presence of a functional occlusion with unrestricted mandibular movements for mild asymmetry cases, then orthognathic surgery is best confined to a camouflage genioplasty
7. With maxillary occlusal cants, an aesthetic judgement must be made based on incisal display, on whether to impact the maxilla on the excess side or downgraft the maxilla on the deficient side regardless of where the aberrant or compensatory growth lies

Timing of corrective surgery

Early surgery (during growth phase)

1. To stimulate development of a functional occlusion through the creation of proper interocclusal relationship at an early age
2. To stimulate soft tissue development on affected side
3. Early aesthetic and functional improvement has a positive psychological effect on both parents and child

Delayed surgery (after growth is completed)

1. Possible untoward effects of early surgery on subsequent facial growth
2. Difficulty in predicting final facial form if early surgery is planned
3. More predictably stable result with less likelihood of multiple procedures

Condylar hyperplasia

Unilateral continued growth of mandibular condyle after completion of skeletal growth. Unknown aetiology–about one-third of patients have a history of trauma.

Clinical

Enlarged condylar process with asymmetrical displacement of mandible away from affected side in both the horizontal and vertical directions resulting in:

1. Posterior open bite – in adults
2. Maxillary occlusal cant – in children where maxilla has compensated for abnormal mandibular growth
3. Scissor bite – shift in dental midlines with crossbite malocclusion on opposite side

Diagnosis

Serial observation over time using:

1. Plain X-rays – including orthopantomograms and cephalograms which may demonstrate an enlarged irregular condyle
2. Models and photos
3. Radioisotopic bone scan

Treatment planning

Must consider:

1. Duration of the condition
2. Evidence of continued growth
3. Evidence of neoplasia, i.e. chondroma
4. Any dental compensations that have occurred

    a. Additional skeletal and dental compensations will need to be corrected by more than just condylectomy due to growth of maxilla, to match abnormal mandibular growth
    b. Where skeletal and dental compensations have not occurred, then condylectomy alone may cure the condition

Treatment

1. Where growth is *continuing* in the adult patient

    - Condylectomy – to eliminate site of aberrant growth followed by correction of deformity after condylar stump has healed

2. Where growth has *ceased*

    - Ramus osteotomy – to shorten the ramus and preserve the functional condyle
    - Bimaxillary surgery – to correct the maxillary occlusal cant

Condylar hypoplasia/agenesis

Unilateral defects

1. Condylar trauma at birth or during early childhood
2. Progressive hemifacial atrophy (Parry–Romberg syndrome)
3. Hemifacial microsomia (Goldenhar syndrome)

Bilateral defects

1. Pierre Robin syndrome – self correcting with time
2. Oto mandibular dysostosis (Treacher-Collins syndrome)

Treatment

During the growth phase

1. Functional appliances
2. Growth centre transplant

    - Costochondral rib

3. Onlay graft

    - To build up tissue bulk at angle of mandible

After completion of growth

1. Mandibular ramus osteotomies

    - Normal side = VSS
    - Hypoplastic side = inverted 'L' with interpositional bone graft in the presence of a satisfactorily functioning TMJ
    - Costochondral rib may be used where there is no functional TMJ

2. Bimaxillary osteotomy ± orthodontics to correct facial asymmetry and occlusal cant

3. Surgical camouflage

   - Onlay graft augmentation to fill in tissue deficiencies
   - Genioplasties to align chin point where occlusion is acceptable

Hemifacial microsomia (craniofacial microsomia)

Clinical features

1. Asymmetrical (unilateral) facial hypoplasia which is present at birth. Sometimes occurs bilaterally hence the term 'craniofacial microsomia' has recently been introduced
2. Aplasia or hypoplasia of mandibular ramus and condyle
3. Hypoplastic malformed ear involving pinna and middle ear deafness
4. Reduced size of maxillary, temporal and malar bones producing flattening of involved side
5. Variable cardiac defects (50% cases) and renal anomalies

Aetiology and pathogenesis

1. 1 in 3500 live births
2. Complex but unknown aetiology, but familial instances do occur suggesting autosomal inheritance

Poswillo (1973) showed in animal models that the severity of the branchial arch dysplasia is related to the degree of haematoma from rupture of the stapedial artery in the region of the ear and jaw during the embryological period of differentiating tissue.

Classification (Pruzansky)

1. Mild deformity – dimunitive but functional TMJ
2. Moderate deformity

   a. Functional but medially displaced dimunative TMJ
   b. Non-functional rudimentary TMJ (condylar stump) and ascending ramus

3. Severe deformity – missing TMJ and ascending ramus

Goldenhar syndrome (oculoauriculovertebral dysplasia)

A varient of hemifacial microsomia with additional vertebral anomalies and epibulbar dermoids

Treatment

During the growth phase

1. Functional appliances – for mild class I cases
2. Growth centre transplant
   - Costochondral rib (moderate class II to severe class III)
   - Microvascular osseomyocutaneous free flap (severe class III)
3. Onlay graft (camouflage)
   - To build up tissue bulk at angle of mandible

After completion of growth

1. Mandibular ramus osteotomies
   - Normal side = VSS
   - Hypoplastic side = inverted ‘L’ with interpositional bone graft in the presence of a satisfactorily functioning TMJ
   - Costochondral rib may be used where there is no functional TMJ
2. Bimaxillary osteotomy ± orthodontics to correct facial asymmetry and occlusal cant
3. Surgical camouflage
   - Onlay graft augmentation to fill in tissue deficiencies
   - Genioplasties to align chin point where occlusion is acceptable

Progressive hemifacial atrophy (Parry–Romberg syndrome)

Progressive unilateral facial atrophy of unknown cause, which first appears in early childhood (< 10 years). The average progress of the disease last for 3 years then becomes static for the rest of life.

Aetiology

Unknown. Previous trauma?, familial?, altered peripheral trophic sympathetic system?

Natural history

1. Atrophy begins in temporalis and buccinator muscle
2. The process then extends to eyebrow, angle of mouth, neck and may even involve half of body

Clinical features

1. Overlying skin is darkly pigmented
2. Atrophy of half of upper lip and tongue is common
3. Enophthalmus – due to loss of periorbital fat
4. Ptosis of eyelid and inability to shut eyes completely
5. Horner's syndrome evident – dilated and fixed pupil
6. Neurological findings:

    a. Trigeminal neuralgia
    b. Facial paraesthesia/weakness/paralysis
    c. Epilepsy is a late occurrence

7. Oral findings:

    a. Body and ramus shorter on involved side
    b. Retarded tooth eruption/atrophic roots

Differential diagnosis

1. Hemifacial microsomia – present from birth, hypoplastic teeth on affected side
2. Scleroderma
3. Fat necrosis

Treatment

Cosmetic augmentation of atrophied side of face involving a combination of skeletal onlay grafting and soft tissue expansion to restore symmetry through bulk.

Hemihypertrophy

First described by Meckel (1822).

Classification (Rowe 1962)

1. Hemifacial hypertrophy
2. Simple hemihypertrophy – single limb affected
3. Complex hemihypertrophy – ipsilateral and/or contralateral sides affected

NB: True or partial hemihypertrophy depends on how much of the body is involved and if all tissues are affected to the same degree.

Aetiology

Congenital – may not be discernible until growth ensues. The process stops with cessation of growth.

Theories put forward

1. Vascular or lymphatic malformations
2. Neurocutaneous lesions
3. Endocrine disorders
4. CNS lesions
5. Disorder of regulative mechanisms at the cellular level during embryological development

Incidence

240 cases reported in the literature upto 1987; 1 in 86 000 US hospital records. Rowe reports M=F.

Clinical features

1. Thickened skin with increased pigmentation
2. Increased bone size with bone defects and digital anomalies
3. CNS – cerebral enlargement, fits and 15–20% mental retardation
4. *Abdominal tumours* — very important to look for this in all cases

   a. Nephroblastoma (Wilms' tumour)

   b. Adrenal cortical carcinoma
   c. Hepatoblastoma

5. Facial involvement

   a. Unilateral enlargement of jaw bones and facial skeleton
   b. Macroglossia with increased size of papillae
   c. Macrodontia with shortened roots, missing or anomalous teeth
   d. Precocious eruption of teeth
   e. Hypercementosis

Histology

1. Increased number of cells and layers in epithelium
2. Increased fibrous connective tissue and prominent vascular channels

Differential diagnosis

1. Hemifacial atrophy – muscle weakness and neurological defects present
2. Fibro-osseous lesions – these cause serum chemistry changes
3. Neurofibromatosis, vascular or lymphatic malformations

Treatment

1. Ultrasound examination of abdomen to exclude neoplasia
2. Emotional support during developing years until growth ceases before surgery can begin
3. Reconstructive surgery

   a. Soft tissue debulking
   b. Face lifts
   c. Ostectomies and osteotomies

Hemimandibular elongation (*Fig. 7.3*)

Refers to a unilateral excessive growth of the mandibular body in the anteroposterior direction.

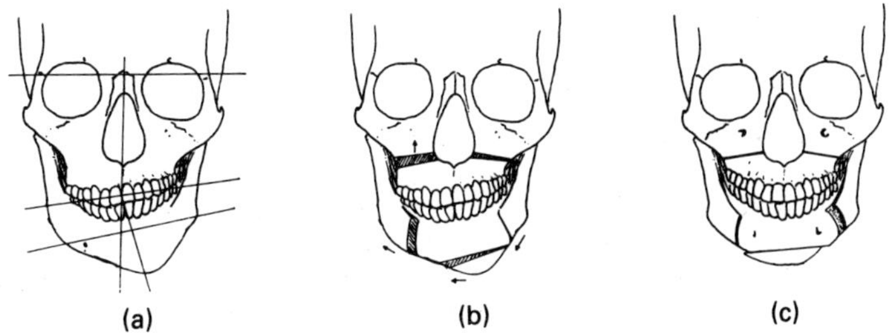

Figure 7.3 Surgical correction of hemimandibular elongation. (a) Skewed mandible with compensatory canted growth in maxilla. (b) Surgical plan – differental maxillary impaction, asymmetrical mandibular shift with propeller type genioplasty. (c) Surgical result.

Clinical features

1. Class III skeletal base tendency of one side of the mandible only (the affected side)
2. Sometimes there may be bowing of the lower border of the affected side of the mandible
3. Teeth on the affected side are of normal size
4. Often this condition will usually present with an elongated or hyperplastic condylar process on the affected side
5. Posterior crossbite or posterior open bite may be present on affected side depending on the degree of compensatory growth of the maxilla

Treatment

1. Mandibular ramus osteotomies in combination with orthodontics as one would do for mandibular AP excess to set-back the mandible on the affected side
2. Where there is bowing of the lower border, then a reduction mandibuloplasty may be warranted

Hemimandibular hypertrophy (*Fig. 7.4*)

Refers to a unilateral excessive growth or enlargement of whole one side of the mandible (including body, ramus, condylar process and *teeth*) in all dimensions of height, width and length.

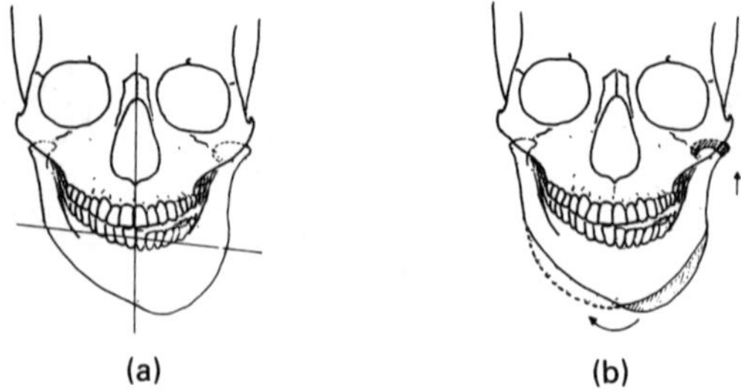

Figure 7.4 Surgical correction of hemimandibular hypertrophy (after Obwegeser). (a) Note the maintenance of dental midlines with unilateral posterior open bite. (b) Surgical procedure – unilateral partial condylectomy and mandibuloplasty with transposition of ostectomized inferior border.

Clinical features

1. It may occur as an isolated entity, i.e. mandible only affected
2. Alternatively, it may form part of a more generalized condition of hemihypertrophy (see previous notes on hemihypertrophy)

Treatment

Debulking procedures such as mandibuloplasty, peripheral ostectomies or shaves aim to reduce overall size of affected mandible.

TMJ ankylosis

Causes of limited mandibular opening (Rowe 1982)

1. Trismus (muscle spasm)

- Myofascial pain and dysfunction
- Submasseteric, temporal space infections
- Mandibular fracture
- Tumours invading masticatory muscles (Trotter's syndrome)
- Tetanus
- Central or peripheral neurological lesions
- Hysterical trismus

2. Pseudoankylosis (mechanical interference)

- Trauma, depressed malar fracture resulting in mechanical obstruction or fibrous adhesions with coronoid process
- Hyperplasia of coronoid process

- Neoplasia of coronoid process
- Scarring of masticatory muscles – myositis ossificans, radiotherapy, submucous fibrosis

3. *False ankylosis (extracapsular in origin)*

a. Trauma

- Periarticular fibrosis (wounds or burns)
- Chronic dislocation of long duration

b. Infection

- Chronic periarticular suppuration (pyogenic/mycotic/TB)

c. Neoplasia

- Fibrosarcoma of capsule (rare)

d. Radiation

- Periarticular fibrosis/osteoradionecrosis
- Inhibition of condylar cellular activity (child)

4. *True ankylosis (intracapsular in origin)*

a. Trauma

- Intracapsular comminuted fracture (especially in child)
- Penetrating wounds (gunshot and/or infected)

b. Iatrogenic

- Previous open surgery for TMJ

c. Infection

- Otitis media/mastoiditis
- Osteomyelitis
- Haematogenous

d. Systemic arthropathy

- Still's disease (juvenile osteoarthritis)

- Ankylosing spondylitis (Marie–Strümpell disease)
- Osteoarthritis
- Rheumatoid arthritis

e. Neoplasia

- Chondroma/osteochondroma/osteoma
- Sarcoma/fibrosarcoma
- Metastases to condyle

f. Miscellaneous

- Chondromatosis (loose bodies)

Sequelae

Child

1. Facial asymmetry – growth stimulus for surrounding tissues is absent due to relative joint inactivity
2. Severe retrognathia – bilateral involvement < 6 years

Adult

1. Inadequate, uninteresting semisolid diet
2. Poor oral hygiene – increased caries and periodontal disease

Basic surgical objectives

Treatment must be commenced as soon as the condition is diagnosed.

1. To establish jaw movement and jaw function
2. To prevent relapse
3. To restore appearance
4. To achieve normal growth and occlusion in the child by interceptive treatment

Perioperative considerations

1. Intubation difficulties

a. Fibreoptic or blind intubation
b. Occasional elective tracheostomy

2. *Children require*

    a. Orthodontic treatment
    b. Growth centre grafts after excision of ankylosis

Surgery for TMJ ankylosis

Osteoarthrotomy

Simple division of bone at the articular surface or condylar neck is seldom indicated because of high incidence of reankylosis.

Osteoarthrectomy

Removal of a block of bone, either the complete condyle (condylectomy) or full thickness section of condylar neck (gap arthroplasty).

- Gap must be as wide as possible because simple osteoarthrectomy, as a result of high recurrence rate, is now rarely performed without some interpositional grafting
- Due to loss of ramus height, some postoperative occlusal derangement occurs and if performed bilaterally an open bite results
- No MMF needed and active jaw movement begun 7 days postoperatively

Osteoarthrectomy and interpositional arthroplasty

Excision of segment of ramus above lingula, leaving ankylosed mass, and deliberate insertion of suitable graft material between new surfaces to prevent bone union. If materials are inserted within periosteal envelope, new bone will grow around this envelope resulting in high recurrence.

Interpositional grafts used

1. Inferiorly based temporalis muscle flap
2. Full thickness skin graft (from abdominal wall)
3. Dermis
4. Cartilage – autogenous (ear), xenograft (bovine)
5. Total joint reconstruction

    a. Costochondral grafts
    b. Microvascularized free grafts
    c. Alloplastic implant or prosthesis (adults)

Coronoidotomies and temporalis myotomies

To help increase mouth opening and is usually recommended at the same time as the ankylosis release.

Adjunctive orthognathic surgical procedures

Where ankylosis of the TMJ occurs during childhood, then lower facial asymmetry is often the resultant sequel, particularly in unilateral cases. Orthognathic surgery plays a significant role in the overall management of these young patients. However, it cannot be undertaken until the first two basic surgical objectives are achieved (i.e. to establish jaw movement and function and to prevent relapse) as described previously.

Treatment aims

Treatment aims of orthognathic surgery in ankylosis cases in children are as follows:

1. Restore normal facial symmetry
2. Achieve a functional occlusion

Treatment

1. Presurgical orthodontics
2. Bimaxillary osteotomy – which should also address the problem of a maxillary occlusal cant
3. Genioplasty – to align the deviated chin point
4. Onlay grafts – may be helpful in building out a deficient mandibular angle projection on the affected side

Note: The difficult part of the orthognathic procedure in ankylosis patients is deciding what ramus osteotomy to perform on the affected side. An inverted 'L' with interpositional bone graft will at least enable an increase in vertical height of the deficient ascending ramus.

Further reading

Bowden CM and Kohn MW (1973) Mandibular deformity associated with unilateral absence of the condyle. *J. Oral Surg.* **31**, 469.

Bruce RA and Hayward JR (1968) Condylar hyperplasia and mandibular asymmetry. *J. Oral Surg.* **26**, 281.

Epker BN and Fish LC (1986) *Dentofacial Deformities: Integrated Orthodontic–Surgical Correction.* CV Mosby, St Louis.

Epker BN and Wolford LM (1980) *Dentofacial Deformities*. CV Mosby, St Louis.

Farkas LG and Cheung G (1981) Facial asymmetry in healthy North American Caucasians. An anthropometrical study. *Angle Orthod.* **51**, 70.

Grayson BH, Boral S, Eisig S *et al*. (1983) Unilateral craniofacial microsomia. *Am. J. Orthod.* **84**, 225.

Obwegeser HL and Makek MS (1986) Hemimandibular hyperplasia–hemimandibular elongation. *J. Maxillofac. Surg.* **4**, 183.

Poswillo D (1973) The pathogenesis of the first and second branchial arch syndromes. *Oral. Surg.* **35**, 302.

Poswillo D (1974) Orofacial malformations. *Proc. Roy. Soc. Med.* **67**, 343.

Poswillo D (1974) Otomandibular deformity: pathogenesis as a guide to reconstruction. *J. Maxillofac. Surg.* **2**, 73.

Poswillo D (1979) Etiology and pathogenesis of first and second branchial arch defects: the contribution of animal studies. In: Converse JM, McCarthy JG, Wood-Smith D (eds): *Symposium on Diagnosis and Treatment of Craniofacial Anomalies.* CV Mosby, St. Louis.

Proffit WR and White RP (1991) *Surgical–Orthodontic Treatment*. Mosby Year Book, St Louis.

Pruzansky S (1975) Anomalies of the face and brain. In: Bergsma D, Langman J, Paul NW (eds): *Morphogenesis and Malformation of the Face and Brain. National Foundation* **11**, 7.

Rowe NL (1962) Hemifacial hypertrophy. *Oral Surg.* **15**, 527.

Rowe NL (1982) Ankylosis of the temporomandibular joint. *J. R. Coll. Surg. Edin.* Part 1: **27**: 67, Part 2: **27**: 167, Part 3: **27**: 209.

Shah SM and Joshi MR (1978) An assessment of asymmetry in the normal craniofacial complex. *Angle Orthod.* **48**, 141.

Souyris F, Moncarz V and Rey P (1983) Facial asymmetry of developmental aetiology: a report of nineteen cases. *Oral Surg.* **56**, 113.

Vig PS and Hewitt AB (1975) Asymmetry of the human facial skeleton. *Angle Orthod.* **45**, 125.

Chapter 8

Principles of grafting and fixation

Introduction

Grafting and fixation play a key role in the stability of orthognathic procedures and hence will be considered together in this chapter. At the present time the most commonly used grafting material in orthognathic surgery is either autogenous bone or a calcium phosphate ceramic such as hydroxyapatite. Currently the most popular form of fixation in orthognathic surgery is rigid internal fixation with plates and screws.

Grafting

Definition

A graft is a substance, foreign to the region of the body in which it is placed, which is used to replace, augment or fill a defect created by surgery, trauma, disease or developmental deficiency.

Types of grafts

1. Autograft – autogenous tissue is procured from and inserted into the same individual
2. Allograft (homograft) – a graft transferred between genetically dissimilar individuals of the same species, i.e. allogenic bone, homologous blood
3. Xenograft (heterograft) – a graft transferred between individuals of different species
4. Isograft – graft transferred between genetically identical individuals (twins or inbred strains)
5. Alloplast – non-biological material

Bone grafts

Requirements of a bone graft

1. Osteogenesis
2. Structure
3. Contour
4. Support
5. Function

Functions

To act as a scaffold for ingrowth of new bone via:

Active process

1. Osteogenesis – to provide a bridge of osteogenic tissue
2. Osteoinduction – active stimulation of osteogensis via osteoblast mitosis

Passive process

1. Osteoconduction – passive invasion of vascular and cellular components of living bone
2. Osteoprotection – to allow the delicate newly-formed woven bone to mature unhindered

Physiology of bone regeneration

Possible sources of osteogenesis

1. Periosteum
2. Osteoblasts

Theories on bone healing

1. Osteoblastic theory (Axhausen 1909)
2. Induction theory (Urist 1956)

Concepts of phased bone regeneration

1. Cellular phase – hours to weeks as proposed by osteoblast theory

2. Induction phase – starts at about 10 days and involves bone morphogenic protein (BMP)

Viability of graft

1. Transplant – a living graft which has the capacity for survival and proliferation after grafting
2. Lyophilized – a devitalized graft (deproteinized, cells removed prior to freeze drying) which no capacity for proliferation after grafting

Ensuring bone graft vitality

1. Recipient graft bed with good blood supply
2. Avoid haematoma and infection
3. Minimize heat production at time of procurement
4. Minimize drying by decreasing delay from procurement to grafting
5. Avoid freezing or boiling

Autogenous bone grafts

Cortical bone

1. Invaded by blood vessels which travel along pre-existing harversian systems
2. Osteoclasts then produce marked porosity within graft which increases liability to fracture
3. All cortical bone graft is eventually replaced after 12 months by resorption and deposition of new bone
4. Usually dies after transplantation as a free graft, resorbs and remodels much slower than cancellous bone grafts
5. Acts as a good mechanical strut

Cancellous bone

1. Early revascularization and cellular activity. Rapidly invaded by woven bone (2 weeks) which eventually resorbs as both the grafted and newly formed bone disappear to make way for development of lamellar bone in 3 months
2. Incorporated into the skeletal tissues of host bone more rapidly than cortical bone

Allogenic bone grafts

Living bone

- Rarely used because they excite an active immune response
- Tissue typing and matching with immunosuppression currently being investigated

Dead bone (bank bone)

- Devitalized by freeze drying, decalcification, lyophilization, irradiation, boiling, or chemical treatment to remove organic material
- Calcining – heating to leave only bone mineral, surface decalcified freeze-dried bone

Improving effectiveness of allogenic bank bone

1. Place the graft in close proximity to living bone of host with either high osteogenic capacity (cancellous bone) or high osteogenic potential (marrow)
2. Myelo-osseous composite allograft–autograft (CAA) = where the allograft bank bone is impregnated with autologous red marrow or cancellous bone of host in order to revitalize and ossify foreign graft
3. Millipore filters (Gortex) – used to isolate graft and only allow cells to pass through to permit revitalization
4. Osteoinduction – chemical or physical factors contained in the allogenic graft, that after contact with connective tissue of the host cause those cells to differentiate into osteoblasts. Tissues which have been shown to be osteoinductors include:

    a. Marrow
    b. HCl decalcified freeze-dried cortical bone

Bone grafting in orthognathic surgery (*Fig. 8.1*)

Indications

Where the gap between the osteotomized segments of bone is large enough to create a substantial likelihood of relapse, then an interpositional bone graft is highly recommended. It is still not clear, however, what the minimum gap dimensions between osteotomized segments is likely to most benefit from grafting, but various recommendations have been made in the literature, often

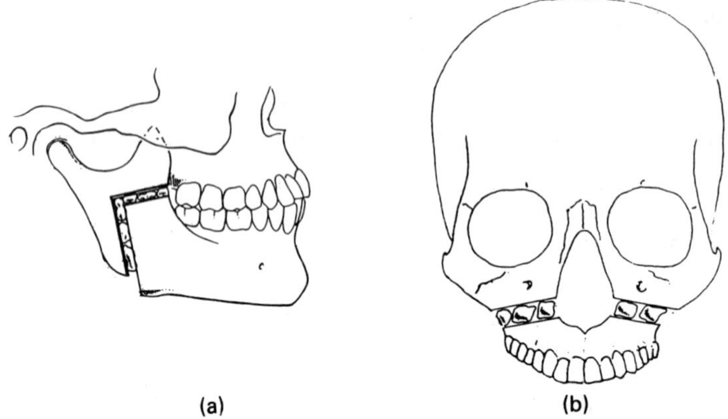

Figure 8.1 Interpositional bone grafting. (a) Inverted 'L' ramus osteotomy. (b) LeFort I maxillary downgraft and advancement osteotomy.

without substantial data. The most common situations where interpositional bone grafts are required are:

1. LeFort I maxillary advancements > 5 mm
2. LeFort I maxillary downgrafts > 3 mm
3. LeFort I maxillary osteotomies in cleft patients
4. Inverted 'L' ramus osteotomies of mandible
5. Vertical augmentation genioplasties
6. Transverse maxillary expansion > 5 mm at any one osteotomy site (not including surgically assisted rapid maxillary expansion procedures)

Most commonly used donor sites

For harvesting of autogenous bone in orthognathic surgery the most commonly used donor sites are:

1. Iliac crest – anterolateral
2. Calvarium – outer table
3. Rib – not as common now
4. Jaws – bone removed during osteotomy is saved and reused as graft

Advantages of autogenous bone grafts

1. Greater healing potential – better quality and quantity of bone formation

2. No immune response elicited
3. No transmission of infectious diseases, i.e. hepatitis or HIV

Disadvantages of autogenous bone grafts

1. Second operative site
2. Increased morbidity

Potential donor site problems

1. Pain
2. Limitation of function – e.g. gait disturbance, adynamic ileus, atelectasis
3. Infection – i.e. seroma, haematoma, wound dehiscence
4. Haemorrhage
5. Contour deformity – e.g. depression in skull vault
6. Unsightly scar – hypertrophic or keloid

Calcium phosphate ceramics

Calcium phosphate biomaterials

Polycrystalline ceramics derived from individual crystals that are fused together by high temperature processes called sintering or hot pressing.

Sintering

Compacting calcium phosphate powders under high pressure into a given shape which is then sintered at temperatures in the range of 1100–1300 °C to produce:

- Hydroxyapatite (HA)
- Tricalcium phosphate (TCP)

Depending on the processing conditions, both dense and porous structures can be produced.

Hot pressing

Compressed and heated simultaneously.

Limitations

Brittle with low impact resistance

- Low tensile strength

Biological profile

Biocompatibility

- No local or systemic toxicity
- No inflammation or foreign body response

Osteogenic potential

Animal studies have shown that calcium phosphate implants are *not* osteoinductive (i.e. do not induce bone formation especially in non-bony tissues). However, they have been shown to be *osteoconductive* (i.e. allow bone ingrowth by serving as a substrate for hard tissue growth).

Autogenous bone grafts heal much faster (4–6 weeks) than calcium phosphate grafts (14–16 weeks).

Porous vs dense hydroxyapatite

Bone growth within the porous structure of HA does not occur since bone proliferates and remodels according to its dynamic environment.

Bone requires some degree of mechanical stimulation to maintain vitality hence it will not grow into unnatural pores, especially pores $< 150\ \mu m$ where the environment is virtually devoid of mechanical stress.

With dense implants, the impervious calcium phosphate particles allow the investing tissues to grow over and around the particles according to environmental influences, i.e. stress.

Types of hydroxyapatite

Solid blocks

Extremely dense. Undergo little/no resorption.

Porous blocks

1. Micropores

    - Pores 1–5 mm, biodegradable

2. Macropores

   - Pores 150–200 mm are optimal for ingrowth of mineralized bone upto 1 mm
   - Minimally biodegradable and strength decreases exponentially with increase in porous size

3. Porous coralline blocks ('Interpore 200')

   - Highly organized and permeable porous structure for ingrowth of lamellar bone
   - Average pore diameter 200 μm
   - Developed by Replamineform technique – hydrothermal treatment which converts reef coral, genus Porites (aragonite $CaCO_3$) to hydroxyapatite $Ca_{10}(PO_4)_6(OH)_2$

Particles

- About 1 mm, used as mouldable implants
- Several forms: irregular and multifaceted, smooth and rounded, irregular surface porosity, regular porous (coralline) structure

Clinical uses of hydroxyapatite in orthognathic surgery

Dense solid blocks

- Dense blocks function as inert and permanent space fillers which enhance stability but provide no osteogenic activity
- Unsuitable in areas subjected to large bending forces because of the high modulus of elasticity

Porous blocks (Interpore 200)

- Allow tissue ingrowth which anchors the implant even in soft tissue
- Easier to cut and shape at the time of surgery but still quite brittle
- Degradation rate of about 2–5% per year

Facial augmentation

- Placed directly on to bone beneath periosteum and fixed with wire or screw
- After 4–6 weeks the implants are permeated by connective

tissue which permanently fixes them in position and prevents migration

Non-porous particles

Not utilized in orthognathic surgery.

Rigid internal fixation (RIF)

The direct fixation of osteotomy sites by plate and screw osteosynthesis.

Advantages of RIF

1. Primary bone healing via
   a. Rigid immobilization
   b. Intimate contact
2. Improved mechanical and functional stability via
   - Greater contact area between bone and screw
3. Direct and precise anatomical reduction
   - No need to distract fracture cleft
4. Less morbidity
   a. No MMF (mandibulomaxillary fixation) required
   b. Rapid return of jaw function and body weight (Cawood 1985)
   c. Better oral hygiene
   d. Less postoperative discomfort

Limitations of RIF

1. Stress shielding. Osteoporosis may develop under the RIF which protects the fracture cleft from the normal functional forces of bone remodelling since forces are mediated via plate which has a higher modulus of elasticity
2. Inflammation
   a. Metal corrosion

   b. Foreign body reaction
   c. Bone resorption around internally stressed appliances

3. Interference – with radiotherapy, CT scans, MRI (*NB*: there is little problem with titanium)

4. Bulk

   a. Patient discomfort, i.e. orbital fractures, which is minimized with microplates
   b. Interference with graft revascularization

5. Expense

Complications with RIF

1. Infection
2. Wound dehiscence

   a. Angle of mandible – where plate is just under incision on external oblique ridge
   b. Delay in treatment
   c. Poor oral hygiene

3. Malocclusion

   a. Associated condylar injuries
   b. Compression osteosynthesis

Precise positioning of osteotomized segments is important with RIF.

4. Sensory disturbance

   a. Placement error – mental nerve, vital teeth
   b. Tissue retraction

5. Delayed/non-union

Failure of RIF

1. Operator inexperience and poor technique
2. Infection

3. Metal fatigue – loose screws, plate fracture
4. Wound dehiscence and exposure – *keep clean and immediate removal is unnecessary*

Removal of RIF

1. Clinical indications

   a. Infection and wound dehiscence
   b. Pain/discomfort

2. Radiographic indications

   a. Bone resorption
   b. Loose or displaced plates/screws

3. Theoretical indications

   - Stress shielding – Cawood 1985, recommends removal after 3 months for miniplates whilst removal of larger fracture plates (AO/ASIF) is recommended after 6 months.

RIF techniques

1. Adaptational

   - Monocortical screws and plates (miniplates, microplates)

2. Compression

   a. Bicortical screws and plates (AO/ASIF)
   b. Lag screws

Rigid internal fixation in orthognathic surgery (*Figs 8.2* and *8.3*)

RIF is now almost exclusively used for almost all orthognathic procedures (except vertical subsigmoid ramus osteotomies). Although RIF has rendered mandibular–maxillary fixation unnecessary, it has nonetheless become common practice to insert light intermaxillary elastics for occlusal guidance and patient comfort postoperatively.

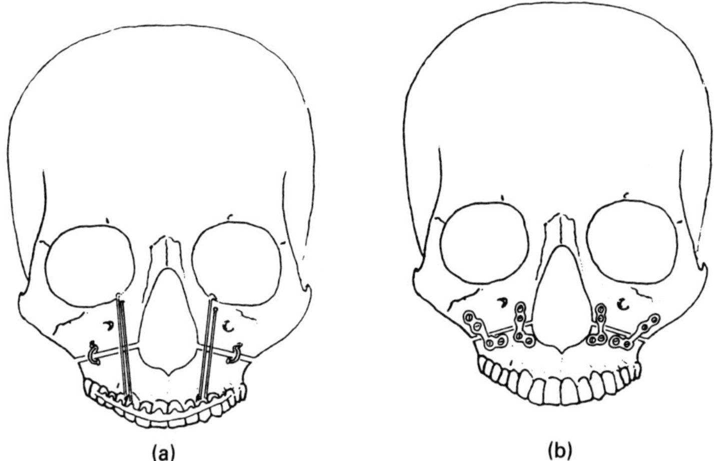

Figure 8.2 Fixation techniques for LeFort I maxillary osteotomies. (a) Transosseous and infraorbital suspension wires. (b) Rigid internal fixation with adaptational plates and monocortical screws.

RIF techniques (see Chapters 4 and 5)

RIF techniques most often used in orthognathic surgery are:

1. Adaptational plates in maxilla (*Fig. 8.2b*)
2. Bicortical screws in sagittal split ramus osteotomies (*Fig. 8.3c* and *d*)
3. Adaptational plates in mandibular osteotomies including sagittal splits (*Fig. 8.3e* and *f*)

Note: Compression techniques for mandibular osteotomies create undesirable shifts in the proximal segments particularly the condyle.

Relapse in relation to RIF

The introduction of RIF in orthognathic surgery has resulted in a flurry of literature particularly focused on the relationship between RIF and relapse. There is little doubt that RIF has served to diminish the incidence of relapse. However, various other factors have been studied and the following conclusions drawn:

1. Self tapping screws are best used in cortical bone 3 mm or less

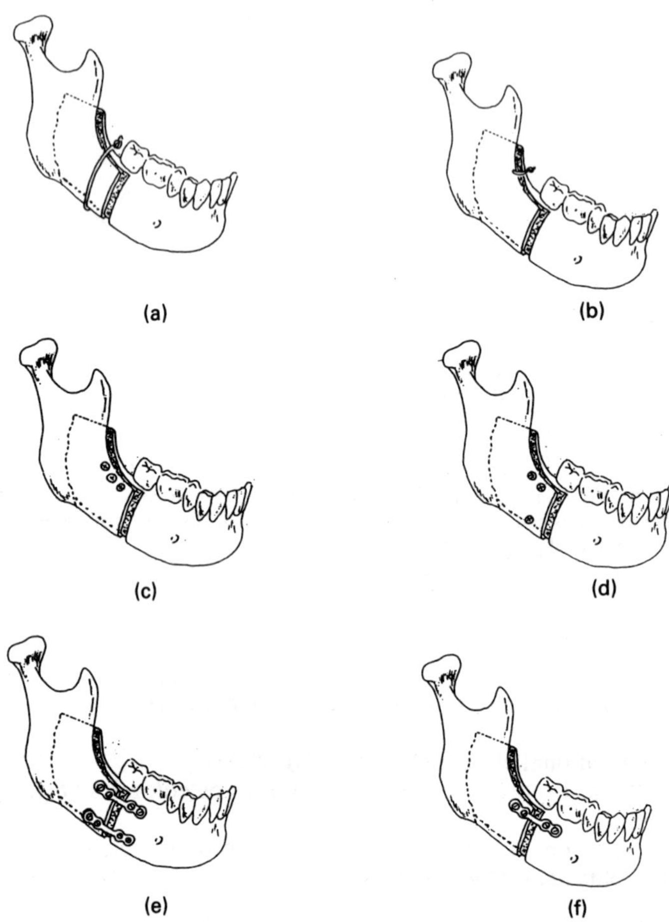

Figure 8.3 Fixation techniques for the sagittal split ramus osteotomy (see Chapter 4). (a) Circumferential wires (rarely used). (b) Transosseous wires (rarely used). (c) Bicortical screws – all in upper border. (d) Bicortical screws – in triangulation pattern (probably the most stable and popular method). (e) Two plates and screws (useful for unfavourable splits). (f) Single upper border plate and screws – for proximal screws may be bicortical.

in thickness and pretapped screws are probably most useful where cortical bone is greater than 3 mm thick

2. There is no difference in holding power between screws placed in the lag or bicortical manner
3. There is no difference in the holding power between screws 2.0 mm thick and 2.7 mm thick

4. In the fixation of sagittal split ramus osteotomies, the triangular pattern of screw insertion with two placed superiorly and one inferiorly at right angles provides the strongest union able to withstand the forces of mastication
5. For very large osteotomy movements the role of RIF in preventing relapse appears somewhat limited and in these cases adjunctive measures such as bone grafting, intermaxillary fixation and skeletal fixation are often employed

Further reading

Araujo A, Schendel SA, Wolford LM *et al*. (1978) Total maxillary advancement with and without bone grafting. *J. Oral Surg.* **36**, 849.

Becker R (1974) Stable compression plate fixation of mandibular fractures. *Br. J. Oral Surg.* **12**, 13.

Block MS and Kent JN (1984) Long term evaluation of hydroxylapatite augmentation of deficient mandibular alveolar ridges. *J. Oral Maxillofac. Surg.* **42**, 793.

Brons R and Boering G (1970) Fractures of the mandibular body treated by stable internal fixation: a preliminary report. *J. Oral Surg.* **28**, 407.

Brons R, Rozema FR, Boering G *et al*. (1990) Bioresorbable osteosynthesis in maxillofacial surgery: present and future. *Oral Maxillofac. Surg. Clin. North Am.* **2**, 745.

Cawood JI (1985) Small plate osteosynthesis of mandibular fractures. *Br. J. Oral Maxillofac. Surg.* **23**, 77.

Champy M, Lodde JP, Jaeger JH and Wilk A (1976) Osteosyntheses mandibulaires selon à technique de Michelet—I. Basesbiomechaniques. *Rev. Stomatol.* **77**, 569.

Champy M, Lodde JP, Schmitt R *et al*. (1978) Mandibular osteosynthesis by miniature screwed plates via a buccal approach. *J. Maxillofac. Surg.* **6**, 14.

Ellis E (1993) Rigid skeletal fixation of fractures. *J. Oral Maxillofac. Surg.* **51**, 163.

Ellis E and Gallo W (1986) Relapse following mandibular advancement with dental plus skeletal maxillomandibular fixation. *J. Oral Maxillofac. Surg.* **44**, 509.

Ellis E and Ghali GE (1991) Lag screw fixation of anterior mandibular fractures. *J. Oral Maxillofac. Surg.* **49**, 13.

Evans AJ, Burwell RG, Merville LC *et al*. (1985) Residual deformities. In Rowe NL, Williams JLl (eds) *Maxillofacial Injuries*. Vol 2, Ch 18, pp 765–868. Churchill Livingstone, Edinburgh.

Keller EE and Triplet WW (1987) Iliac bone grafting: review of 160 consecutive cases. *J. Oral Maxillofac. Surg.* **45**, 11.

Leonard MS (1990) Rigid internal fixation: facts versus fallacies. *Oral Maxillofac. Surg. Clin. North Am.* **2**, 737.

Marx RE (1993) Philosophy and particulars of autogenous bone grafting. *Oral Maxillofac. Surg. Clin. North Am.* **5**, 599.

Paulus GW and Steinhauser EW (1982) A comparative study of wire osteosynthesis versus bone screws in the treatment of mandibular prognathism. *Oral Surg. Oral Med. Oral Pathol.* **54**, 2.

Persson G, Hellem S and Nord PG (1986) Bone plates for stabilizing LeFort I osteotomies. *J. Maxillofac. Surg.* **14**, 69.

Powell NB and Riley RW (1987) Cranial bone grafting in facial aesthetic and reconstructive contouring. *Arch. Otol Head Neck Surg.* **113**, 713.

Souyris F (1978) Sagittal splitting and bicortical screw fixation of the ascending ramus. *J. Maxillofac. Surg.* **6**, 198.

Spiessl B and Schroll K (1972) Gesichtsschadel. In: Nigst H (ed): *Spezielle Frakturen Und Luxationslehre*. Vol 1. Georg Thieme Verlag, Stuttgart.

Spiessl B (1989) *Internal Fixation of the Mandible. A Manual of AO/ASIF Principles*. AO/ASIF, Berlin.

Steinhauser EW (1982) Bone screws and plates in orthognathic surgery. *Int. J. Oral Surg.* **11**, 209.

Terjesen T, Nordby A and Arnulf V (1986) The extent of stress protection after plate osteosynthesis in the human tibia. *Clin. Orthop. Rel. Res.* **207**, 108.

Tucker M, Terry W, White R and Van Sickels JE (eds) (1990) *Rigid Fixation for Maxillofacial Surgery*. Lippincott, Philadelphia.

Urist MR and McClean FC (1952) Osteogenic potency and new bone formation by induction in transplants to the anterior chamber of the eye. *J. Bone Joint Surg.* **34A**, 443.

Urist MR (1956) Bone formation by autoinduction. *Science* **150**: 983.

Urist MR, Silverman B, Buring K *et al.* (1967) The bone induction principle. *Clin. Orthop.* **53**, 243.

Urist MR and Strates BS (1971) Bone morphogenic protein. *J. Dent. Res.* **50**, 1392.

Wardrop R and Wolford L (1989) Maxillary stability following downgraft and/or advancement procedures with stabilization using rigid fixation and porous block hydroxyapatite implants. *J. Oral Maxillofac. Surg.* **47**, 336.

Wolford LM, Wardrop RW and Hartog JM (1987) Coralline porous hydroxylapatite as a bone graft substitute in orthognathic surgery. *J. Oral Maxillofac. Surg.* **45**, 1034.

Zins J and Whitaker L (1983) Membranous vs endochondral bone: implications for craniofacial reconstruction. *Plast. Reconstr. Surg.* **72**, 778.

Zins J, Kusiak J, Whitaker L and Enlow DH (1984) Influence of recipient site on bone grafts to the face. *J. Plast. Reconstr. Surg.* **73**, 371.

Chapter 9

Adjunctive cosmetic surgery

Introduction

General principles

1. There must be an overall 'balance' of individual facial components that will fit well in a given patient's face (*Figs 9.1* and *9.2*)
2. Racial and ethnic variations must be considered
3. Generally, orthognathic surgery must be completed first prior to any planned adjunctive cosmetic procedure, which may be perfomed in the same operation or staged at later date as a secondary procedure

The nose in orthognathic surgery

Applied surgical anatomy of the nose

1. *Neurosensory innervation*

   a. Nasal skin

   - Infraorbital nerve – lateral aspect
   - Infratrochlear nerve – nasal bridge
   - Anterior ethmoidal nerve – nasal tip

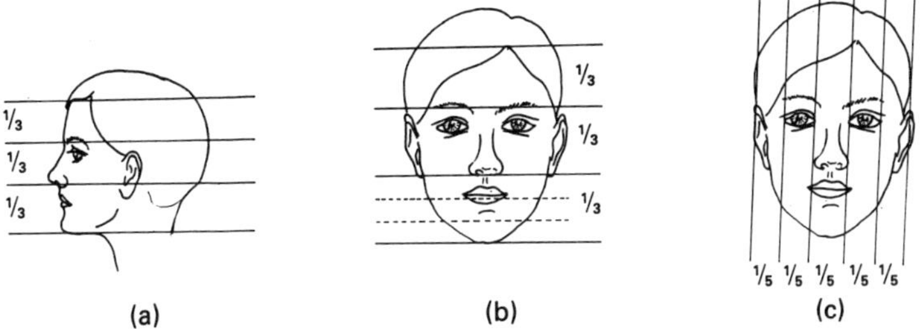

Figure 9.1 Aesthetic facial proportions. (a) Facial thirds in profile. (b) Frontal view of facial thirds. (c) Vertical facial fifths.

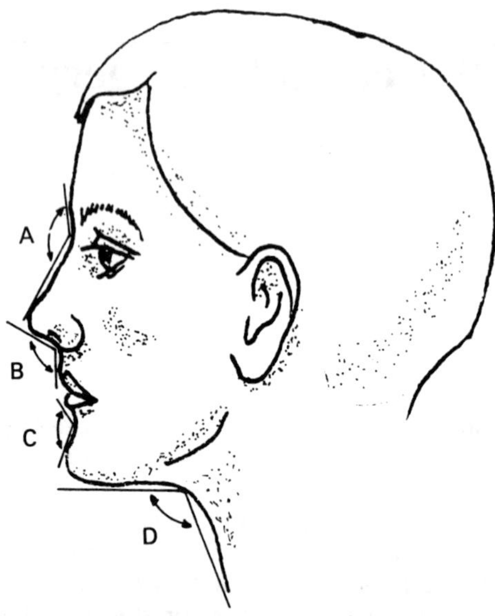

Figure 9.2 Important clinical facial angulations. A, frontonasal angle; B, nasolabial angle; C, labiomental fold; D, chin–throat angle.

b. Lateral nasal wall

- Anterior ethmoidal nerve – anteriorly
- Posterior inferior and superior nasal branches of descending palatine nerve

c. Nasal septum

- Anterior ethmoidal nerve
- Nasopalatine nerve

2. Vascular supply

Branches from the facial artery (externally), ethmoidal, palatine and sphenopalatine arteries (internally).

3. Soft tissue coverage

a. The soft tissue coverage is thickest over the nasal tip and thinnest over the dorsum; in the latter it is much harder to camouflage irregularities of the bony osteotomies
b. Muscle coverage over the nose includes procerus and

corrugator muscles superiorly over the root of the nose and muscles of the nasalis group laterally and inferiorly

c. Two muscular aponeurotic systems:
   i. Nasal – superficial
   ii. Perichondrial – deep

4. *Hard tissues*
   a. Bones
      i. External – paired nasal bones, frontal process of maxilla
      ii. Internal – ethmoid, maxilla, inferior concha
      iii. Septum – perpendicular plate of ethmoid, vomer
   b. Cartilage
      i. Internal – septal
      ii. External – upper lateral, lower lateral (alar)

Clinical aesthetic evaluation of nose

1. *Basic aesthetic nasal components*
   a. Radix – root of the nose (nasal bridge)
   b. Dorsum
   c. Tip
   d. Columella
   e. Nares
   f. Alar base
2. *Perspectives*
   a. Frontal
   b. Profile
   c. Three-quarter oblique
   d. Basal
3. *Objective parameters*
   a. Symmetry – e.g. nares
   b. Projection – e.g. of nasal tip
   c. Width – e.g. alar base
   d. Angle – e.g. nasolabial

Rhinoplasty technique

Objectives

1. Aesthetics
2. Function – combined with septoplasty and turbinal surgery to improve nasal airway

Methods

1. Closed rhinoplasty – subcutaneous method of modifying the nasal skeletal framework which relies heavily on tactile rather than the visual sense of the surgeon
2. Open rhinoplasty – where the nasal skeletal framework is exposed for direct visual access to the operative site

Basic steps of rhinoplasty

The classic steps in rhinoplasty as listed below in sequence must be adapted to each individual case, hence not all the steps may be required. Through an understanding of the changes incurred with each step, the rhinoplasty is adapted to the individual characteristics of the nose.

1. Anaesthesia – under sedation or endotracheal general anaesthesia the nose is packed with cocaine soaked gauze then infiltrated with a vasoconstrictor containing local anaesthetic solution
2. Skeletonization of nasal framework – via an intercartilagenous incision
3. Tip-plasty and nasal shortening
4. Hump removal and profile lowering
5. Narrowing of the nose – the nasal osteotomies
6. Splinting and intranasal packing – 4–7 days

Indications for open rhinoplasty

More time consuming than closed procedures. However, the following relative indications for the open approach have been cited:

1. Secondary cleft nose
2. Crooked or asymmetric nose
3. Revision rhinoplasty

4. Difficult nasal tip deformities
5. Teaching of rhinoplasty technique

Rhinoplasties and orthognathic surgery

Timing

1. Delayed – rhinoplasty performed after orthognathic surgery
2. Simultaneous – rhinoplasty performed at the same operation as orthognathic surgery

Delayed rhinoplasties

Rationale

Reasons for avoiding simultaneous jaw and nasal surgery:

1. Compromised potential airway
2. Inability to reliably judge nasal aesthetics intraoperatively
3. Avoids a lengthy operation and hence minimizes postoperative morbidity
4. More accurate assessment of changes in nasal aesthetics after orthognathic surgery
5. Allows resolution of trauma to nasal mucosa resulting from maxillary osteotomy

Simultaneous rhinoplasty with orthognathic surgery

Rationale

Reasons for combining jaw and nasal surgery at the same operation.

1. Patient convenience – eliminates the need for a second operation
2. Improved access – for septal and turbinate surgery (improve nasal airway) with a LeFort I downfracture
3. Take advantage of the predicted favourable nasal changes that occur with maxillary surgery, e.g. enhance tip projection when maxilla is impacted or advanced
4. Corrects or prevents unfavourable nasal changes during maxillary surgery, e.g. alar cinch to control flaring of alar base with maxillary advancement

Indications

1. Where mandibular surgery and/or genioplasty is performed without maxillary surgery
2. Where maxillary surgery is considered careful patient selection is strongly advised; the only two situations where results can be accurately predicted in conjunction with maxillary osteotomies are:

    a. Large dorsal humps
    b. Broad noses

Limitations

With the LeFort I maxillary osteotomy, minor nasal deformities are best managed with a delayed rhinoplasty since surgical manipulation of the septum, anterior nasal spine and soft tissues of the lip as well as the maxillary base in a maxillary osteotomy can produce a profound and at times unpredictable change in the nasal tip and nasolabial angle.

Furthermore, since the maxillary osteotomy is undertaken first, the tissue oedema and altered nasal morphology will cloud the surgeon's judgement as to final outcome of the rhinoplasty.

Patients should always be informed about the possibility of revision surgery.

The neck in orthognathic surgery

Reasons for a poorly aesthetic neck

1. Laxity of soft tissues – excess skin folds usually in the aged
2. Lipomatosis – excessive adipose tissue
3. Mandibular retrognathia
4. Microgenia – where the chin flows into the neck
5. *Iatrogenic* – in the presence of existing or potential fullness in the neck the following orthognathic procedures will worsen the aesthetics:

    a. Mandibular set-back
    b. Reduction genioplasty
    c. Maxillary downgraft (inferior positioning)

Surgery for the unaesthetic neck

The type of surgery required depends on the underlying reason(s) for the neck deformity hence:

1. Lipectomy – most useful in cases of lipomatosis in young people where the contours of the neck are obliterated by localized accumulation of adipose tissue. There are various lipectomy procedures, viz:

   a. Suction lipectomy – where there is good skin elasticity
   b. Transoral lipectomy – where there is fat deep to platysma
   c. Open transfacial lipectomy – with platysma muscle plication, skin excision or both. Used for correction of chin ptosis as well as removal of mild redundant skin

2. Rhytidectomy (facelift) – most effective where there is a moderate to severe laxity of redundant soft tissues

3. Orthognathic surgery – mandibular advancements and/or appropriate genioplasties will address the problem of an unaesthetic neck related to mandibular deficiency

Suction lipectomy of cervical mandibular (submental) area

Gaining popularity as a valuable and simple adjunctive procedure for many orthognathic cases.

Equipment

Blunt ended cannulas with non-cutting openings attached to high airflow vacuum pump with filter and collection bottles.

Procedure

1. Best if patient is in sitting position when marking out areas of fat to be removed
2. Cannula is introduced through a 6–8 mm midline submental incision that is further opened up by blunt dissection with scissors into the fat layer
3. A No. 4 or 6 cannula is inserted into the correct tissue plane with the cannula opening facing away from the skin
4. The vacuum is turned on and multiple passes are made with the cannula in the areas marked out for fat removal, taking care to leave an even thickness of subcutaneous fat attached to the skin
5. An area from the mentum to the inferior aspect of the mandibular angle can be approached through the submental incision

6. The thickness of the remaining fat is assessed by pinching and rolling the skin with fingers and thumb
7. Apply pressure to express fluid and blood before primary closure with 6/0 synthetic suture
8. Elastic support pressure dressing applied for 5–7 days; thereafter a night dressing is worn for 2–3 weeks. Analgesia is prescribed

Complications

Apart from pain and ecchymosis, post-operative sequelae are few in experienced hands. However, the following potential complications may arise:

1. Haematoma, seroma – infection
2. Skin dimpling, waviness, depressions and adherence to underlying tissues – where fat removal is uneven
3. Poor case selection or inadequate treatment planning (i.e. concomitant treatment of dentofacial deformity not treated) can lead to poor results

Simultaneous orthognathic and cosmetic neck surgery

Cosmetic neck procedures are best undertaken after the completion of orthognathic surgery but preferably at the same operation, unless a facelift is indicated in which case it is best undertaken as a secondary procedure at a later date.

Types of simultaneous procedures commonly performed

1. Mandibular set-back with suction lipectomy
2. Genioplasty with transoral lipectomy – utilize the same incision for access
3. Transfacial lipectomy, skin excision ± platysma plication may be performed with any orthognathic procedure where there is redundant skin

The cheeks in orthognathic surgery

The aesthetic components of a cheek

1. Cheek proper
2. Paranasal region
3. Buccal region

Clinical assesment

Important features to look out for are:

1. Asymmetry
2. Degree of prominence*
3. Degree of deficiency*

*In relation to surrounding facial landmarks.

Patient must be evaluated from different perspectives, i.e. frontal, profile, basal, three-quarter oblique.

Surgical augmentation of cheeks

1. Alloplastic implants – most common procedure, whereby implant may be custom prefabricated prior to operation or sculptured intraoperatively
   a. Hydroxyapatite
   b. Other – *NB* Silastic and Proplast–Teflon have raised serious concerns about long-term biocompatability and adverse tissue reactions
2. Onlay grafts – resorption is common
   a. Autogenous bone – rib, ilium, cranial
   b. Cartilage
   c. Fat and collagen
3. Osteotomies – complex procedures with high morbidity and unpredictable results
   a. Zygomatic complex
   b. High LeFort osteotomies, e.g. quadrangual LFII, LeFort III, etc.
4. Combination
   - e.g. LeFort I maxillary osteotomy with alloplastic cheek implants

Further reading

Beeson WH and McCollough EG (1986) *Aesthetic Surgery of the Aging Face*. CV Mosby, St Louis.

Bernstein L (1975) Surgical anatomy in rhinoplasty. *Otolaryngol. Clin. North Am.* **8**, 549.
Epker BN and Stella JP (1990) Systematic aesthetic evaluation of the neck for cosmetic surgery. *Oral Maxillofac. Surg. Clin. North Am.* **2**, 217.
Epker BN and Stella JP (1990) Simultaneous orthognathic and cosmetic neck surgery. *Oral Maxillofac. Surg. Clin. North Am.* **2**, 259.
Kennedy BD (1990) Suction lipectomy of the youthful neck. *Oral Maxillofac. Surg. Clin. North Am.* **2**, 233.
Kennedy BD (1990) Adjunctive procedures in maxillofacial surgery. *Oral Maxillofac. Surg. Clin. North Am.* **2**, 795.
Powell NB, Riley RW and Laub DR (1988) A new approach to the evaluation and surgery of the malar complex. *Ann. Plast. Surg.* **20**, 206.
Sheen J (1987) *Aesthetic Rhinoplasty*. CV Mosby, St Louis.
Waite P, Matukas V and Sarver D (1988) Simultaneous rhinoplasty procedures in orthognathic surgery. *Int. J. Oral Maxillofac. Surg.* **17**, 298.
Waite PD (1990) Simultaneous orthognathic surgery and rhinoplasty. *Oral Maxillofac. Surg. Clin. North Am.* **2**, 339.
Wisth PJ (1975) Nose morphology in individuals with angle class I, II, or III occlusions. *Acta Odont. Scand.* **33**, 53.

Chapter 10

Orthognathic surgery in special cases

Introduction

Orthognathic surgery plays a significant and important role in the overall management of the following conditions. Each condition entails specific requirements for which the orthognathic surgical technique is readily adapted to with some occasional minor modifications.

1. Cleft lip and palate
2. Post-traumatic facial deformities
3. Preprosthetic surgery
4. Obstructive sleep apnoea
5. Temporomandibular disorders
6. Tumour surgery

Cleft lip and palate

Incidence

- 1:650 or 1.7 per 1000 live births
- Cleft lip – more common in males (2:1)
- Cleft palate – more common in females
- Racial predilection – mongoloid > caucasian > negroid

Classification

- Primary palate (right and left)

  i. Lip
  ii. Alveolar process

- Secondary palate

  i. Hard palate
  ii. Soft palate

Group 1

Clefts involving *primary* palate, i.e. lip and/or alveolus.

Group 2

Complete clefts involving *primary* and *secondary* palates, i.e. lip, alveolus, hard palate, soft palate.

Group 3

Clefts involving *secondary* palate, i.e. hard palate, soft palate (submucous cleft).

- Bifid uvula
- Muscle diastema
- Notch in hard palate

Importance of cleft treatment

Anxiety and frustration related to :

- Poor appearance
- Speech impairment
- Hearing loss
- Feeding difficulties – nasal regurgitation
- Adverse attitudes of parents, peers and society

which ultimately affect personality and behaviour of the child as well as their assimilation into society, i.e. poor schooling and job prospects.

Secondary deformities

Deformities that arise as a result of growth and surgical intervention. Banks (1983) – the fundamental problems of repaired clefts are:

1. Absent or hypoplastic tissues – resulting from embryonic deficiency and diminished growth potential
2. Misplaced hard and soft tissues – resulting from inadequate or incomplete primary or interceptive surgery
3. Deformity – resulting from the effects of scar tissue produced by interceptive surgery during development

Treatment of clefts

Team approach

Complete rehabilitation calls for a co-ordinated multidisciplinary treatment:

1. Dental – oral and maxillofacial surgeon, orthodontist, prosthodontist, paedodontist
2. Medical – paediatrician, plastic surgeon, ENT surgeon
3. Paramedical – speech therapist, psychologist, social worker

Stages in cleft lip and palate treatment

1. 1–4 weeks	Parental counselling, presurgical infant orthopaedics (seldom used)
2. 8–12 weeks	Lip repair
3. 12–18 months	Palatal repair*
4. 6–11 years	Speech therapy
5. 7–14 years	Orthodontic treatment
6. 8–11 years	Alveolar cleft bone grafting*
7. 9–19 years	Pharyngoplasty, grommets
8. 17–19 years	*Orthognathic surgery* Lip revision, rhinoplasty Fixed prosthodontics Social and vocational counselling
9. Adult	Closure of oronasal fistula Preprosthetic surgery, i.e. vestibuloplasties Removable prosthodontics

*There is much controversy concerning the timing of these procedures depending on which school of thought one adheres to.

Surgical management of cleft lip and palate

Primary surgery

1. Lip repair
2. Palatal repair

Secondary surgery

1. Lip

    - Removal of scar tissue

- Correction of vermillion border
- Obicularis muscle reconstruction

2. Nose

- Straighten and lengthen columella
- Normalize alar base and nares

3. Palate

- Closure of oronasal fistulae

4. Alveolus (*Fig. 10.1*)

- Bone grafting
- Vestibuloplasty to deepen sulcus

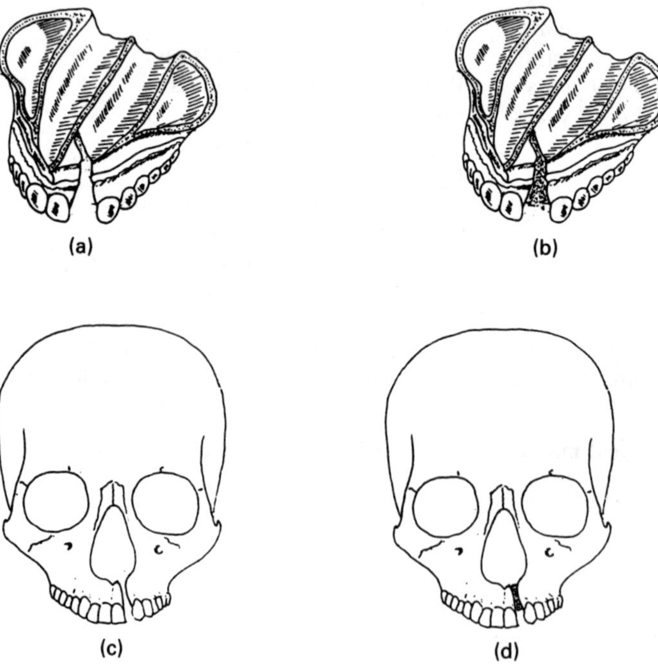

Figure 10.1 Secondary bone grafting of alveolar clefts. (a) and (b) View of maxilla before and after bone grafting. (c) and (d) Facial skeletal view of alveolar cleft deformity before and after bone grafting.

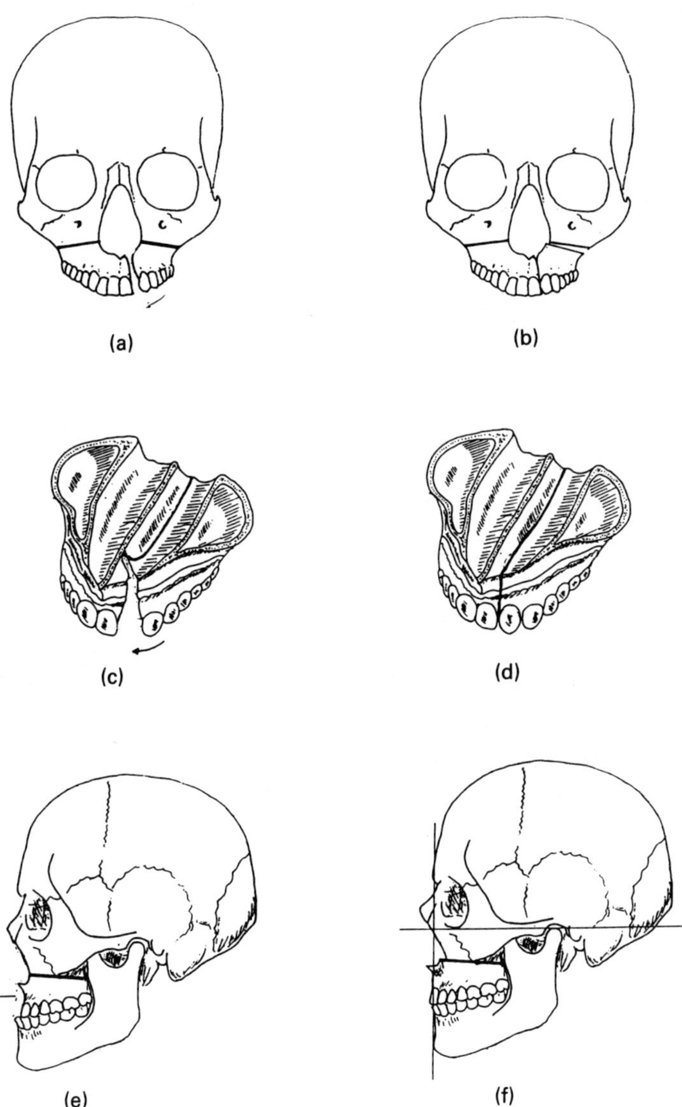

Figure 10.2 Management of alveolar cleft with orthognathic surgery. (a) LeFort I osteotomy with segmental maxilla. (b) Lesser segment rotated medially to close cleft defect. (c) Downfractured maxilla showing alveolar cleft defect. (d) Lesser segment osteotomized and advanced and rotated medially to close alveolar cleft defect, with canine in lateral incisor position. (e) Lateral skull view of cleft palate patient showing horizontal (AP) hypoplasia of maxilla with relatively normal mandible. (f) Surgical result after LeFort I maxillary advancement.

5. *Jaws* (*Fig. 10.2*)

    - *Orthognathic surgery*

6. Velopharyngeal incompetence

    - Pharyngoplasty

Objectives in reconstruction of secondary cleft deformities

1. Nose and upper lip – the most frequent presenting complaint; of significant aesthetic concern to the patient
2. Midfacial hypoplasia – in both anteroposterior and vertical dimensions
3. Occlusion – orthognathic surgery, orthodontics, restorative dentistry and prosthetics
4. Oronasal fistulae and alveolar defects

    - Air and fluid leakage
    - Anterior bone deficiency
    - Poor denture retention and lack of sulcus depth
    - Deficient osseous support for teeth

5. Speech – surgery must not further compromise poor speech

Orthognathic surgery

Cleft dentofacial deformity

1. Pseudo-class III malocclusion

    - Hypoplastic maxilla
    - Normal mandible

2. Anterior open bite – posterior crossbites

Timing of orthognathic surgery

There is a high relapse rate in patients with osteotomies done < 16 years old. Therefore, if early jaw osteotomies are indicated for psychosocial reasons, then a second orthognathic procedure at a later stage should be anticipated.

Recommendation – best to undertake orthognathic surgery after completion of growth (males 18 years old; females 17 years old).

LeFort I maxillary advancement (*Fig. 10.2*)

The most commonly performed osteotomy for cleft patients.

Surgical design and approach

1. Dictated by the nature of the cleft, i.e. unilateral or bilateral

    a. Unilateral clefts – osteotomy same as for non-clefts
    b. Bilateral clefts – premaxilla remains attached to pedicle of vestibular mucosa

2. Compromised palatal blood supply from previous surgery necessitates vertical vestibular incisions with subperiosteal tunnels
3. Scar tissue within cleft area must be completely removed to allow complete mobilization of all maxillary segments

Surgical limitations

1. Maxillary advancement may accentuate velopharyngeal incompetence. May require delayed pharyngoplasty
2. Maxillary advancement limited by:

    a. Previous pharyngoplasty
    b. Scarred upper lip

3. Rigid fixation provides good horizontal stability but poor vertical stability

Adjunctive procedures

1. Presurgical orthodontics. Rapid maxillary expansion
2. Alveolar grafting – facilitates surgery by allowing en bloc movement of the whole maxilla, although it has no role in postoperative stability of maxillary advancement. Usually undertaken 6–12 months prior to maxillary osteotomy. Grafting has also been reported to be done at the same time as osteotomy

Other orthognathic procedures for clefts

1. Bimaxillary surgery – only in severe cleft deformities. Vertical relapse becomes less noticeable

2. LeFort II and III osteotomies – used in total midface hypoplasia or where poor palatal blood supply prohibits the use of the LeFort I advancement
3. Segmental maxillary osteotomies (*Fig. 10.2*)

   a. Unilateral clefts

      - Major and minor segments
      - Advancement or lateral rotation
      - Alone or in combination

   b. Bilateral clefts

      - premaxilla and lateral maxillary segments moved individually or simultaneously. Premaxilla is mobilized with a substantial labial pedicle

4. Mandibular set-back osteotomy – in combination with onlay grafting to deficient maxilla. Mandibular surgery is best reserved for cases where maxillary osteotomies in difficult cleft cases will worsten marginal velopharyngeal incompetence or where maxilla cannot be sufficiently advanced due to scarring

Other considerations

Nasal reconstruction

Nasal deformity

- Some degree of hypoplasia of the alar cartilages may be present
- Alveolar defects have a fundamental effect on the symmetry of nasal shape
- Nasal septum deviates towards the non-cleft side

Surgical objectives

Rhinoplasty should only be done *after* reconstruction of the maxillary base including the alveolar defects. Involves correction of:

1. AP deficiency of nasal sill and tip
2. Asymmetrical nostrils and base
3. Septoplasty to improve airway obstruction

Speech impairment

Primary speech defects

- Velopharyngeal incompetence
- Nasal escape

Secondary speech defects

- Hearing loss – no functional dilatation of pharyngotympanic tube
- Functional muscle weakness
- Poor skills due to psychosocial factors
- Orofacial defects

Speech therapy

Establishing new responses with muscle exercises for improving:

1. Velopharyngeal competence
2. Tongue placement

Speech therapy more effective after surgery and dental treatment has been undertaken.

Orthognathic surgery

- Maxillary advancements will exacerbate speech defect
- Pharyngeal flaps will limit the amount of maxillary advancement to about 5 mm
- If $>$ 5 mm advancement in maxilla is desired, then the existing pharyngeal flap must be divided then surgically redone at a later stage (approx 6–12 months after orthognathic surgery)
- Alternatively on very large maxillary movements the mandible will have to be set-back with an advancement genioplasty to mask the procedure

Post-traumatic facial deformities

Aetiology of maxillofacial injuries

1. Assault
2. Motor vehicle accidents
3. Recreational incidents – contact sports
4. Industrial accidents
5. Falls – children, elderly, epileptics
6. Other – tooth extractions, pathological fractures

Management of maxillofacial injuries

1. Observe – non-displaced or minimally displaced fractures particularly in cases of:

   a. Extremes of age – very old or very young
   b. Patients with terminal prognosis
   c. Severly compromised medical status

2. Closed reduction

   a. No fixation – malar lift via a Gillie's temporal approach
   b. Dental fixation – mandibular–maxillary fixation (MMF) with wires, arch bars, cast metal splints or acrylic 'gunning' splints
   c. External fixation – craniomaxillary frames and pins, mandibular biphasic pins
   d. Internal pin fixation – k-wires

3. Open reduction with internal fixation (ORIF)

   a. Transosseous wires
   b. Adaptational plates and monocortical screws – miniplates, microplates
   c. Compression plates and bicortical screws
   d. Lag screws

Post-traumatic facial deformities

Refers to the resultant facial form after healing of sites of injury is complete. Post-traumatic facial deformities may arise from:

1. Misdiagnosis – fracture sites missed on initial treatment
2. Poor reduction of fractured segments – malunion

3. Inadequate fixation across fracture sites
4. Prolonged delay in definitive management – where fracture sites have healed

Orthognathic surgery

The role of orthognathic surgery in the management of post-traumatic facial deformities is to restore original facial form and function. Presurgical orthodontics is not often required since the fundamental aim is to re-establish the pre-injury status of the patient rather than to create a new environment for the dento-facial complex.

1. Treatment planning is based on:

   a. Patient desires and expectations – probably the most important!
   b. Pre-injury records – i.e. photos, dental charts
   c. Nature of the original injury – clinical records and investigations from institution or practitioner(s) involved in the primary management of the patient's maxillofacial injuries
   d. Treatment subsequently received for the maxillofacial injuries in question
   e. The existing deficiency in form and function that has resulted since the injury

2. Surgery – the surgical procedure may be undertaken in one of two ways:

   a. Recreate old fracture sites – whereby the osteotomies follow the original fracture pattern to refracture and reset the bone fragments to their original pre-injury position. This can be difficult especially for midface fractures whereby the fracture sites are often comminuted
   b. Conventional osteotomies – whereby conventional orthognathic techniques are used at sites not necessarily involving the original fracture(s), e.g. a sagittal split ramus osteotomy is used to correct a post-traumatic deformity resulting from a displaced condylar process fracture that was originally treated by closed reduction

Note: Orthognathic surgery for post-traumatic cases is often technically more difficult to undertake as a result of the extensive scarring and presence of hardware from the original treatment that should, if at all possible, be removed at the same time.

Preprosthetic surgery

Preprosthetic surgical goals

1. To facilitate the construction of a dental prosthetic appliance
2. To secure a stable denture base in order to:

   - Simplify design and construction
   - Enhance retention
   - Counteract displacing forces
   - Reduce the rate of adverse bone and soft tissue changes

Preprosthetic surgical techniques

Alveolar ridge augmentation is one area of preprosthetic surgery where orthognathic surgical techniques may be used. Listed below is range of alveolar ridge augmentation procedures available with orthognathic techniques listed under the heading of 'osteotomies'.

1. Relative augmentation (soft tissues) – where the denture bearing area is increased without an actual increase in the height of the bony alveolus. Example – vestibuloplasty

   a. Secondary epithelialization
   b. Pedicled mucosal grafts
   c. Free grafts, e.g. skin or mucosa

2. Absolute augmentation (hard tissues) – increase in the height of the bony alveolus

   a. Bone grafts

      i. Onlay
      ii. Interpositional

   b. Osteotomies

      i. *Mandible (visor, sandwich)*
      ii. *Maxilla (palatal, segmental, total)*

   c. Alloplastic

      i. Hydroxyapatite

ii. Dental implants

- Endosseous (Branemark)
- Transosseous (Bosker)
- Subperiosteal

NOTE: With the success of endosseous implants, other alveolar augmentation procedures are not as commonly used now. However, onlay grafts to support implants are sometimes employed in selected cases.

Augmentation of maxilla

Orthognathic surgery for maxillary alveolar bone deficiency

1. Palatal vault osteotomy
2. Anterior maxillary osteotomy
3. Total maxillary osteotomy

Palatal vault osteotomy

Indications

- Poor palatal vault but adequate ridge height
- In conjunction with interpositional grafts to improve vault forms
- Improve stability of maxillary prosthesis
- Pseudoaugmentation of the atrophic ridge

Contraindications

- Scarred palate of cleft patient

Disadvantages

- Poor blood supply to palatal segment
- Stability and long-term results unknown

Surgical technique

- Palate is freed by sectioning nasal septum
- Cartilage and bone are removed from the nasal septum to allow for superior repositioning of the palatal bone

Anterior maxillary osteotomy

Indications

- Severe anterior atrophy
- Poor anterior palatal form hence creation of better vault form
- May not require secondary soft tissue procedure
- Total ridge atrophy
- Redundant soft tissue over adequate basal bone

Disadvantages

- Stability unknown

Surgical technique

- Similar to an anterior segmental maxillary osteotomy performed on dentate patients
- Interpositional bone grafting is required

Total maxillary osteotomy

a. Advancement and downgrafts

Indications

- Severe bony deficiency with adequate palatal vault form
- Mild to moderate AP and transverse discrepancies

Contraindications

- Poor palatal vault form

Advantages

- Stable predictable movements
- Changes of ridge relations possible in three dimensions

Disadvantages

- Secondary donor site
- May require vestibuloplasty

Surgical technique

- LeFort I osteotomy with downfracture

b. Palatal vault elevation

- Similar to LeFort I downfracture
- Palatal osteotomy is completed from above whilst maxilla is downfractured
- The palatal segment is detached from rest of maxilla and superiorly repositioned whilst the rest of the maxilla is downgrafted

Augmentation of mandible

Orthognathic surgery for mandibular bone deficiency

1. Visor osteotomy (*Fig. 10.3a*). The cranial fragment is separated by a sagittal (vertical) osteotomy and moved vertically upwards in a sliding fashion
2. Sandwich osteotomy (*Fig. 10.3b*). The cranial fragment is separated by a horizontal osteotomy which is carried out between the two mental foramina. Thus it lifts only the anterior fragment
3. Combination – sandwich/visor. The osteotomy posterior to the mental foramina is in the vertical plane, changing to 45 degrees in the anterior region

The raised cranial fragment is supported by interposed grafts such as autogenous, freeze-dried or alloplastic bone or cartilage.

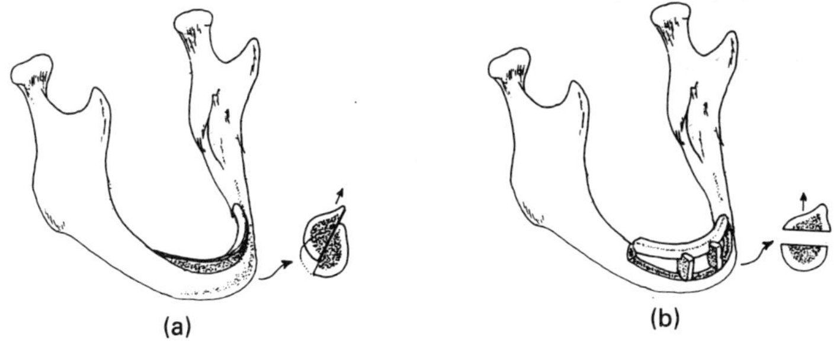

Figure 10.3 Preprosthetic osteotomies for the management of atrophic edentulous mandible. (a) Visor osteotomy. (b) Sandwich osteotomy.

Follow-up

- Fairly stable result expected after initial loss of height in the first 6 months
- Loss of augmented height after 2 years ranges from 28 to 49%
- Collapse of fragments due to pressure from stretched mucosa
- Early vestibuloplasty (< 6 months) compromises blood supply
- Remodelling of 'sharp' cranial segment contributes to loss in height

Complications/limitations

- Nerve damage – 92% after 1 year
- Fracture of atrophic mandible

4. Anterior osteotomy with posterior onlay graft

Objectives

To achieve results similar to the modified visor osteotomy but with less nerve trauma.

Surgical technique

a. Crestal incision beginning from 1 cm behind the mental foramen to the opposite side
b. Subperiosteal tunnel is created posteriorly where blocks of hydroxyapatite are placed as onlay grafts secured with circummandibular wires
c. Anteriorly, between the mental foramena a horizontal osteotomy is performed and alveolar segment is (pedicled on lingual soft tissues) elevated with interpositional allogenic bone grafts
d. Double layered closure

Follow-up

- Vestibuloplasty combined with the lowering of the floor of mouth procedure which may be performed 6 months later
- Long-term results are still uncertain

Obstructive sleep apnoea

Pathogenesis

Electromyograms and video pharyngoscopy have shown that the muscular atonis that develops in the upper airway during sleep can result in collapse or obstruction during inspiration.

It is now generally accepted that there are several areas of excessive redundant tissue such as soft palate, base of tongue and pharyngeal walls of hypopharynx that can contribute to the obstructive process.

Consequences

1. Sleep fragmentation – which manifests as excessive daytime sleepiness
2. Hypoxaemia – which produces hypertension and cardiac arrhythmias

Sites of obstruction

Type 1 Oropharynx
Type 2 Oropharynx–hypopharynx
Type 3 Hypopharynx

Presurgical evaluation

1. Physical examination
2. Fibreoptic pharyngoscopy
3. Cephalometric analysis
4. Polysomnography – to document sleep-related breathing abnormalities using a variety of tests

Surgical management

1. *Tracheostomy*. An early method used to bypass the upper airway, but has turned out to be an undesirable form of treatment from a psychological aspect
2. *Uvulopalatopharyngoplasty (UPPP)*. A modification of a procedure used to correct snoring. The aim is to remove excessive redundant tissue from the posterior soft palate and lateral pharyngeal wall. Several studies have reported a success rate of no more than 50%, because the base of tongue was found to be the cause of continued obstruction

3. *Nasal continuous positive airway pressure (CPAP)*. A non-surgical technique which uses a mask, valve and pressure generator to pneumatically maintain upper airway patency. Its success is dependent on patient compliance which is found to be 65% after 5 months
4. *Orthognathic surgery*. Based on the concept that the position of the base of tongue is dictated by the position of the mandible and hyoid bone. Hence surgical advancement of the mandible and hyoid bone will result in expansion of the hypopharyngeal airway

    a. Hyoid advancement and suspension – hyoid is suspended anteriorly and superiorly to mandible with fascia lata harvested from the thigh (several surgeons use braided suture)
    b. Anterior mandibular osteotomy and hyoid suspension – to advance the position of the tongue also
    c. Mandibular advancement osteotomy – sometimes with maxillary advancement to enable larger advancement of the mandible (*Fig. 10.4*)

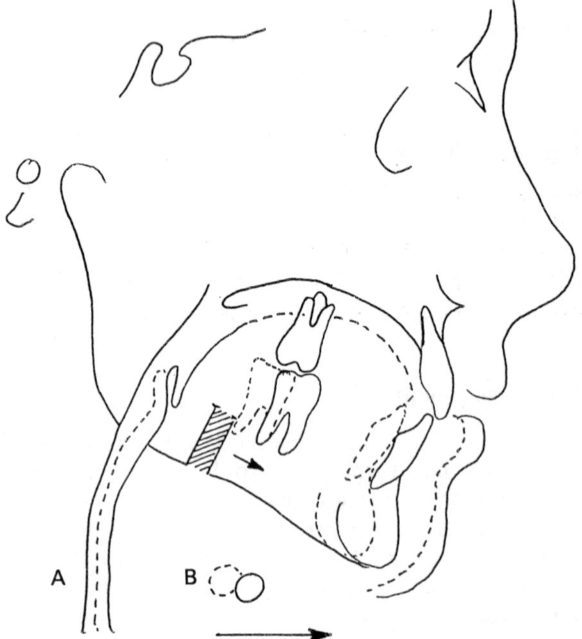

Figure 10.4 Mandibular advancement for the management of obstructive sleep apnoea. A, hypopharyngeal airway; B, hyoid bone; ----, before; ——, after.

d. Total subapical mandibular osteotomy – for class I cases where the dentoalveolar segment is first set-back to class II relationship prior to advancement of whole mandible some months later

Riley *et al*. (1990) treated 40 patients with obstructive sleep apnoea using orthognathic surgery and claimed a 97% success rate. Their indications for orthognathic surgery were severe obstructive sleep apnoea, morbid obesity and severe mandibular deficiency.

Temporomandibular disorders

Temporomandibular disorders (TMD) is a collective term used to describe a number of related conditions that involve the temporomandibular joint (TMJ), masticatory musculature and associated structures which present with many common symptoms such as facial pain and limited mouth opening.

Cardinal features of TMD

1. Pain – most common complaint but the most difficult problem to assess
2. Joint noises – clicking, grating (crepitus). In the absence of pain, its clinical significance is of little importance
3. Restricted jaw function – limited range of mandibular movements in the vertical, protrusive and lateral directions. Also includes inability to chew
4. Other non-specific symptoms – headaches, earaches, tinnitus, neck and shoulder pains, etc.

Clinical evaluation of TMD

1. History

By far the most important component of the overall evaluation. The history may involve the following procedures:

a. Questionnaire – of chief complaint(s) which the patient fills out prior to consultation
b. Visual analogue scales – for degree of pain and chewing ability
c. Pain diagram – where the patient can diagramatically outline site and extent of pain

d. Consultation – during which the clinician elicits the following information from the patient:

   i. Chief complaint(s) – pain, joint noises, restricted joint function, etc.
   ii. Background – duration and detailed nature of symptoms. Chronological history of previous treatments and outcome
   iii. Medical history – allergies, medication, illnesses, operations
   iv. Associated features – stress, depression, anxiety, significant life events, sleep disturbance, bruxism, reliability as a historian, patient expectations, etc.

2. *Clinical examination*

a. Facial symmetry and skeletal pattern – dolicofacial, brachyfacial, etc.
b. Palpation – to elicit tenderness in TMJ or muscles of mastication
c. Assess maximum mandibular range of motion – vertical, protrusive and lateral excursions
d. Deviation on mandibular opening or closing
e. Joint noises – auscultation, palpation
f. Dental and skeletal occlusion – distribution of tooth contact, centric occlusion–centric relation discrepancy
g. Wear facets on teeth – evidence of bruxism

3. *Investigations*

Investigations for the most common TMD such as myofascial pain and dysfunction play a relatively minor role, since the majority of the pertinent information should already have been provided by the history and physical examination. The most useful role for investigations is therefore to eliminate the possibility of less common pathological processes such as ankylosis or neoplasia that may mimic TMD symptoms. The most commonly performed investigations are as follows:

a. Plain radiographs – orthopantomograms, transcranial projection of TMJ; limited to demonstrating any gross bony pathology only
b. CT scans – poor for soft tissue components of TMJ
c. Magnetic resonance imaging – has superseded arthrograms for delineation of disc integrity and position. Very expensive!

d. Arthroscopy – limited to visualization of upper joint space only; also therapeutic

Differential diagnosis

The two most common TM disorders can be identified by the following characteristics:

Myofascial pain and dysfunction (MPD)

1. Pain is cyclic and diffusely distributed in multiple sites in the head and neck
2. Pain is frequently worse in the morning and patient will often report sore teeth from clenching
3. Wear facets on teeth
4. Restricted range of mandibular movements with abnormal jaw posturing
5. Chewing on one side as an avoidance mechanism to sore tooth
6. Occasional large centric relation–centric occlusion discrepancy

Internal derangement

1. Continuous pain which is exacerbated by jaw function
2. Pain is well localized to TMJ
3. Mechanical interferences such as clicking or locking may result in deviation of mandibular movements on opening and closing
4. Decreased range of mandibular movements due to mechanical interferences and sometimes pain

Note: MPD often coexists with internal derangement.

Treatment planning

The treatment schedule selected should aim to alleviate the pain, adverse joint loading, restore mandibular function, reduce or eliminate joint noise and allow the patient to return to normal daily activities. A well designed treatment plan should not only focus on the TMJ or muscles of mastication, but should also attend towards eliminating all contributing factors that serve to maintain or nurture the disease process. This includes the concomitant management of dentofacial deformities that may exist.

Treatment of temporomandibular disorders

It is well established from the literature that over 80% of patients with TMD respond favourably to conservative measures. The remaining 20% are refractory cases that include those with chronic pain syndrome complicated by multiple contributing factors. Approximately 5% of all TMD patients undergoing treatment will require surgical intervention.

Non-surgical treatment

- Explanation and reassurance
- Home exercises
- Medications
- Physiotherapy
- Occlusal therapy – appliances, occlusal adjustments, restorative dentistry
- Behavioural management – biofeedback
- Psychiatric

Surgical treatment

- Arthrocentesis and lavage with manipulation
- Arthroscopy
- Arthrotomy (open joint surgery)
- Modified condylotomy (*Fig. 10.5*)

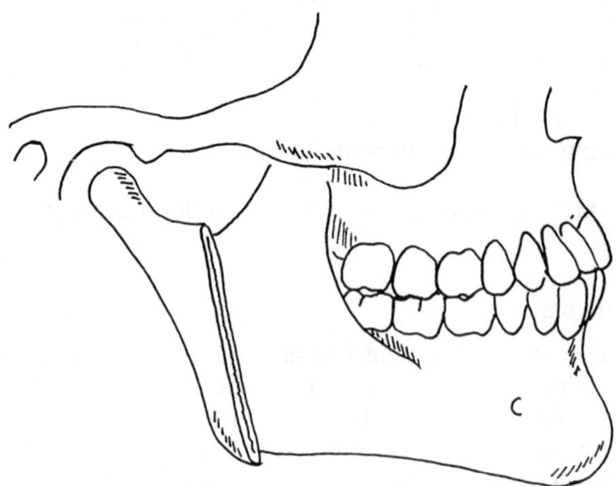

Figure 10.5 Modified condylotomy for the treatment of internal derangement of the temporomandibular joint (after Nickerson).

Relationship between dentofacial deformities and temporomandibular disorders

Dentofacial deformities and malocclusions may lead to adaptive structural changes within the TMJ which occur through altered biomechanical loading of the joints. Hence orthognathic procedures such as a maxillary impaction may alter the biomechanics sufficiently to alleviate TMD symptoms.

The literature appears to show some association between some malocclusions such as skeletal class II deformities, posterior crossbites and anterior open bites. However, such malocclusions are considered as exacerbating factors rather than aetiological factors, in patients who are predisposed to temporomandibular disorders. It is impossible to determine or predict whether orthognathic surgery will lead to a resolution of a temporomandibular disorder in any individual case.

Studies to date have been unable to demonstrate any significant difference in temporomandibular disorders between treated and untreated dentofacial deformities.

Concomitant dentofacial deformity and TMD

Diagnostic evaluation

A clinician must be totally aware of the multiple problems a patient may present with, that may or may not be related. One combination is that of TMD with a concomitant dentofacial deformity. A thorough clinical evaluation of each problem must be performed in order to establish the correct diagnosis. Chapter 2 outlines the evaluation of orthognathic patients and this section has an outline of the clinical evaluation of patients with TMD.

Developing a problem list and prioritizing treatment

When developing a treatment plan for a patient with TMD and dentofacial deformity, the most important first step is to address the patient's chief complaint. Obviously, symptoms of pain should take priority in management over a malocclusion.

Treatment sequence – in TMD/orthognathic patients

1. Manage the TMD. The first step is to control the symptoms of TMD such as pain and muscle spasm through non-surgical means
2. Commence presurgical orthodontics once TMD symptoms are

under control, making certain that regular follow-ups and TMD treatment is maintained during the course of orthodontic treatment

3. Orthognathic surgery. This is best undertaken before any TMJ surgical plan is developed, because it is found that about 90% of patients with TMD and dentofacial deformities improve after orthognathic surgery, and about 10% remain the same or get worse (White and Dolwick 1992). In difficult TMD cases, orthognathic planning should involve, where possible, vertical subsigmoid osteotomies with a period of MMF to enable some enforced period of rest for the joint in addition to treating the internal derangement as one would do using the modified condylotomy technique (Hall *et al*. 1993) (*Fig. 10.5*)
4. TMJ surgery. After orthognathic surgery, the status of the TMD is evaluated and if symptoms of pain and limited mouth opening remain severe and refractory to further non-surgical therapy, then TMJ surgery may be indicated, provided the TMD is not myofascial pain and dysfunction

Simultaneous orthognathic and TMJ surgery

This is not recommended for the following reasons;

1. Lengthy surgery
2. Joint swelling as a result of surgery makes control of occlusion difficult. Simultaneous orthognathic surgery and TMJ arthroscopy or surgery should be discouraged because precise placement of the bony segments is dependent on an accurate condyle–fossa relationship
3. Prolonged MMF if required, may be deleterious to an operated TMJ

Tumour surgery

The techniques of orthognathic surgery may be applied to tumour ablative surgery as a means of establishing direct access to deep seated tumours.

Basic principle

The aim is to establish adequate access without sacrificing bone so that primary bone healing is achieved with minimal postoperative morbidity in terms of functional and cosmetic deformities.

Must apply rigid internal fixation across proposed osteotomy site *prior* to completing osteotomy so that fragments can be accurately relocated to their original relationship at the end of the tumour ablation.

Examples of osteotomies used for access

1. *Anterior mandibulotomies* – linear or stepped, used in combination with lip and tongue splitting incisions for access to posterior third of tongue lesions (*Fig. 10.6a*)
2. *Ramus osteotomies* – particularly the 'VSS' used for access to the parapharyngeal spaces for tumours of the deep lobe of the parotid gland (*Fig. 10.6b*)
3. *LeFort I maxillary downfracture* – with palatal split, used to gain direct access to posterior pharynx, clivus and base of middle cranial fossa
4. *Other variations*

   a. Facial osteoplastic flap – where the whole maxilla, pedicled on a cheek flap, is disarticulated from the rest of the facial skeleton and swung laterally to reveal the post-nasal space
   b. Temporal approach (*Fig. 10.7*) – via a coronal incision, the zygoma is osteotomized and swung inferiorly pedicled on masseter muscle, whilst the coronoid pedicled to temporalis muscle is swung superiorly to establish direct access to the retromaxillary or infratemporal space.

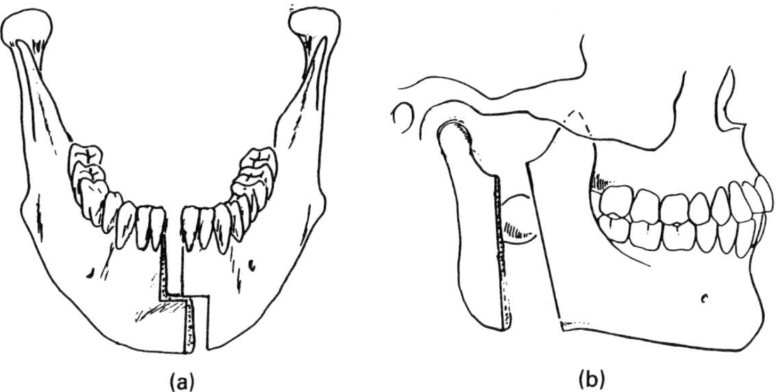

Figure 10.6 Surgical access to deep seated tumours utilizing orthognathic surgical techniques. (a) Stepped anterior mandibulotomy for base of tongue lesions. (b) Vertical subsigmoid osteotomy for access to parapharyngeal tumours.

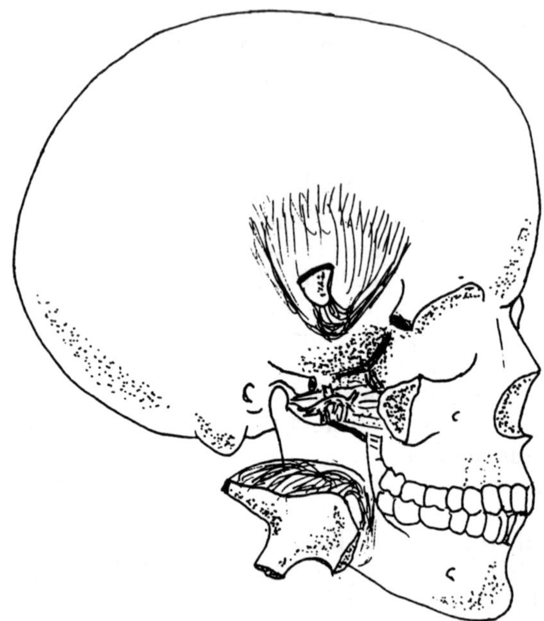

Figure 10.7 Temporal approach to retromaxillary, infratemporal and posterior orbital tumours (after Obwegeser). Note the detached zygoma pedicled on masseter and reflected inferiorly with coronoid pedicled on temporalis and reflected superiorly to expose retromaxillary space.

Further reading

Altemir HF (1986) Transfacial access to the retromaxillary area. *J. Maxillofac. Surg.* **14**, 165.

Banks P (1983) The surgical anatomy of secondary cleft lip and palate deformity and its significance in reconstruction. *Br. J. Oral Maxillofac. Surg.* **21**, 78.

Dolwick MF (1989) Clinical diagnosis of temporomandibular joint derangement and myofascial pain and dysfunction. *Oral Maxillofac. Surg. Clin. North Am.* **1**, 1.

Dolwick MF and Sanders B (1985) TMJ internal derangement and arthrosis: Surgical atlas. CV Mosby, St Louis.

Droukas B, Lindee C and Carlsson GE (1985) Occlusion and mandibular dysfunction: a clinical study of patients referred for functional disturbances of the masticatory system. *J. Prosthet. Dent.* **53**, 402.

Evans AJ, Burwell RG, Merville LC *et al*. (1985) Residual deformities. In: Rowe NL and Williams JLI (eds): *Maxillofacial Injuries*. Vol 2, Ch 18, pp. 765–868. Churchill Livingstone, Edinburgh.

Fonseca RJ and Davis WH (1986) *Reconstructive Preprosthetic Oral and Maxillofacial Surgery*. WB Saunders, Philadelphia.

Grabb WC, Rosenstein SW and Bzoch KR (1979) *Cleft Lip and Palate.* Little, Brown, Boston.

Grime PD, Haskell R, Robertson I and Gullan R, (1991) Transfacial access for neurosurgical procedures: an extended role for the maxillofacial surgeon—I. The upper cervical spine and clivus. *Int. J. Oral Maxillofac. Surg.* **20**, 285.

Grime PD, Haskell R, Robertson I and Gullan R (1991) Transfacial access for neurosurgical procedures: an extended role for the maxillofacial surgeon—II. Middle cranial fossa, infratemporal fossa and pterygoid space. *Int. J. Oral Maxillofac. Surg.* **20**, 291.

Helfrick JF (1991) Treatment of secondary cleft deformities: orthognathic surgery. *Ann. R. Aust. Coll. Dent. Surg.* **11**, 244.

Laskin DM, Ryan WA and Greene CS (1986) Incidence of temporomandibular symptoms in patients with major skeletal malocclusions. *Oral Surg. Oral Med. Oral Pathol.* **61**, 537.

McNeill C (ed) (1993) *Temporomandibular Disorders – Guidelines for Classification, Assessment and Management*. 2nd ed. Quintessence Books, Chicago.

Obwegeser HL (1969) Surgical correction of small or retrodisplaced maxillae. *Plast. Reconstr. Surg.* **43**, 351.

Obwegeser HL (1969) Temporal approach to the TMJ, the orbit, and the retromaxillary infracranial region. *Head Neck Surg.* **7**, 185.

Ochs MW, LaBanc JP and Dolwick MF (1990) The diagnosis and management of concomitant dentofacial deformity and temporomandibular disorder. *Oral Maxillofac. Surg. Clin. North Am.* **2**, 669.

Powell NB and Riley RW (1990) Obstructive sleep apnoea: orthognathic surgery perspectives, past, present and future. *Oral Maxillofac. Surg. Clin. North Am.* **2**, 843.

Proffit WR and White RP (1991) *Surgical–Orthodontic Treatment*. Mosby Year Book, St Louis.

Riley RW, Powell NB and Guilleminault C (1990) Maxillary, mandibular and hyoid advancement for treatment of obstructive sleep apnoea: a review of 40 patients. *J. Oral Maxillofac. Surg.* **48**, 20.

Ross RB (1987) Treatment variables affecting facial growth in complete unilateral cleft lip and palate. Part 1. Treatment affecting growth. *Cleft Palate J.* **24**, 5.

Semb G (1991) A study of facial growth in patients with bilateral cleft lip and palate treated by the Oslo CLP team. *Cleft Palate J.* **28**, 22.

Stoelinga P, Haers P, Leenen R *et al.* (1990) Late management of secondarily grafted clefts. *Int. J. Oral Maxillofac. Surg.* **19**, 97.

Upton LG and Sullivan SM (1990) Modified condylotomies for management of mandibular prognathism and TMJ internal derangement. *J. Clin. Orthod.* **24**, 697.

White CS and Dolwick MF (1992) Prevalence and variance of temporomandibular dysfunction in orthognathic surgery patients. *Int. J. Adult Orthod. Orthognath. Surg.* **7**, 7.

Chapter 11

Craniofacial surgery

Introduction

Through the pioneering efforts of Paul Tessier and others during the 1960s, craniofacial surgery has become almost a routine procedure based on three decades of experience since craniofacial surgery first became a recognized superspecialty. It involves the surgical correction of complex congenital and acquired deformities involving the cranium, orbits, facial bones and jaws. At present craniofacial surgery is performed by teams in only a few major centres worldwide. Because of the complex nature of the problem that craniofacial surgery has to address, a team of specialists headed by a craniofacial surgeon is required to deal with each case.

Principles of craniofacial surgery

1. The facial skeleton remains viable even if stripped of all its periosteum, hence it is possible to expose the whole cranio-maxillofacial complex without detriment to the subsequent healing process
2. With the exception of the orbital foramena, the whole cranio-maxillofacial complex can be osteotomized and moved in any direction
3. The bitemporal (coronal) flap is the most commonly utilized access for all intracranial and most subcranial procedures

Indications

1. Congenital deformities – present at birth
2. Developmental deformities – arising after birth
3. Aquired deformities

   a. Trauma
   b. Disease – neoplastic/non-neoplastic

Timing

Advantages of early surgery (during growth phase)

1. To stimulate soft tissue development around affected areas
2. Early aesthetic and functional improvement has a positive psychological effect on both parents and child
3. Decompression of the intracranial space to reduce intracranial pressure in order to:

   a. Prevent visual problems
   b. Permit normal mental development

4. Achievement of satisfactory craniofacial form to correct an unusually shaped head and face so as to:

   a. Promote peer acceptance and normal assimilation into society
   b. Permit normal psychological and behavioural development

5. Infants are better able to tolerate major surgery due to vastly greater healing potential
6. The problem of restricted airway in cases of severe maxillofacial retrusion has to be promptly addressed

Disadvantages of early surgery

1. Possible untoward effects of early surgery on subsequent facial growth
2. Difficulty in predicting final facial form if early surgery is planned
3. More predictably stable result with less likelihood of relapse and multiple procedures if surgery is performed at the end of growth
4. Blood loss and fluid balance can be difficult to monitor and adequately control especially with major surgery in small infants

Factors which have contributed to advances in craniofacial surgery

1. Excellent healing potential of the craniofacial skeleton
2. Innovative surgical techniques and instrumentation
3. Advances in paediatric anaesthesia techniques
4. Advances in radiological techniques, e.g. 3D CT scans

Craniofacial deformities

Malformation – primary structural defect resulting from a localized error of morphogenesis.
Syndrome – two or more abnormalities in the same individual.
Anomalad – a malformation together with its subsequent derived structural changes.
Sequence – where one condition leads to the next and then the next and so forth.

Importance of diagnosing a syndrome

1. To anticipate other abnormalities that potentially occur with each syndrome so as to alert the clinician of more serious abnormalities
2. To understand the natural history
3. To establish recurrence risk of each particular disorder

Syndromes associated with specific facial deformities

Cleft lip and palate

1. Pierre Robin syndrome
2. Treacher-Collins syndrome (otomandibulofacial dysostosis)
3. Apert's syndrome

Facial asymmetry

1. Hemifacial atrophy (Parry–Romberg syndrome)
2. Hemifacial microsomia (Goldenhar syndrome)
3. Hemifacial hypertrophy
4. Neurofibromatosis (von Recklinghausen's disease)

Midface deficiencies

1. Craniosynostoses

    a. Apert's
    b. Crouzon's
    c. Pfeiffer

2. Binder's syndrome
3. Achondroplasia dwarf
4. Cleidocranial dysplasia

Mandibular deficiencies

1. Pierre Robin syndrome
2. Treacher-Collins syndrome (otomandibulofacial dysostosis)
3. Hemifacial microsomia (Goldenhar syndrome)

Mandibular prognathism

1. Gorlin – Goltz syndrome
2. Osteogenesis imperfecta
3. Marfan syndrome
4. Klinefelter syndrome

Role of orthognathic surgery in craniofacial deformities

Orthognathic surgery must be tailored to the growth pattern of each individual. Importantly, it must consider the growth potential of the patient and target those regions where growth is undesirable. It is generally unknown to what degree early craniofacial surgery affects subsequent facial growth. From studies on cleft patients, the degree of restricted growth after surgery appears to depend on the stage of development of the child at the time of the primary surgery and the amount of tissue manipulation and subsequent scarring that takes place.

Orthognathic surgery often has a significant role in the late management of patients with craniofacial deformities. In the craniosynostoses, patients usually develop a class III skeletal base malocclusion which often requires bimaxillary osteotomies in combination with orthodontic treatment in late adolescence. The branchial arch deformities are somewhat more complex and usually require some form of interventional orthognathic surgery during the early growth phase with a high likelihood of further orthognathic surgery in late adolescence.

Craniofacial deformities often harbour abnormal cephalometric landmarks, making surgical planning on cephalometric prediction tracings somewhat difficult. Hence data collected from clinical examination and dental casts play an even more important role in the formulation of an orthognathic surgical treatment plan.

Craniosynostosis

Definition and types

Deformed shape of skull caused by premature fusion of sutures. 0.4–1 per 1000 live births. About 5% have congenital heart defects.

1. Dolichocephalic – long skull caused by premature fusion of sagittal suture, 55–60% cases. Mental retardation in approx 10% cases
2. Brachycephalic – short skull caused by bilateral fusion of coronal suture, 20-30% cases. Mental retardation in 25% cases
3. Plagiocephaly – skewed cranium caused by unilateral fusion of either coronal or lambdoid suture
4. Turricephaly – pinhead shape caused by premature closure of all sutures
5. Trigonocephaly – where the forehead is shaped like a ship's bow, due to premature closure of metopic suture. Hypotelorism is a common feature

Aetiology

Unknown, probably genetic. About 8% of cases of coronal synostosis and 2% of sagittal synostosis are familial.

Differential diagnosis

Other causes of cranial vault deformity include:

1. Rickets
2. Hypophosphatasia
3. Cranial moulding

Diagnosis

1. Measurement of head dimensions (cephalic index)
2. Lack of movement of calvarial bones in infancy and palpable ridging

Apert's syndrome

Clinical features

1. Turribrachycephaly – with high (steep) flat frontal and occipital bones
2. Hypertelorism – with strabismus and proptosis of eyes
3. Midface hypoplasia – with high arched, constricted palate, anterior open bite, vertical maxillary deficiency and severe malocclusion. A third of cases have cleft of the soft palate

4. Syndactyly (fusion) of fingers and toes – with the bones of the hands, feet and cervical spine becoming progressively synostosed (fused)
5. Mental retardation – in most cases

Aetiology

Unknown. Autosomal dominant inheritance. Increased paternal age at time of conception has been found. 1 in 2 000 000 in general population due to high neonatal mortality.

Prognosis and treatment

Prognosis depends on the degree of mental retardation.

1. Orthopaedic surgery – to correct syndactyly of fingers. Toes are usually not treated
2. Craniomaxillofacial surgery – see below

Crouzon's syndrome (*Fig. 11.1*)

Clinical features

1. Variable and progressive craniosynostosis – usually begins first year of life and progresses to second or third year. Steep forehead with flat occiput and short and narrow cranial base. Seizures in 10% cases
2. Exophthalmus – secondary to shallow orbits. Poor vision in 45% cases
3. Hypoplastic maxilla – narrow high arched palate with open bite and severe dental crowding in upper arch. Ectopic eruption of first molars in upper arch in 50% cases. Short upper lip with drooping lower lip. Beak-like nose
4. Conductive hearing loss – due to malformed ear ossicles in over 50% cases
5. Upper airway obstruction – deviated nasal septum may result in cor pulmonale

Aetiology

Unknown. Autosomal dominant transmission. Increased paternal age may be important.

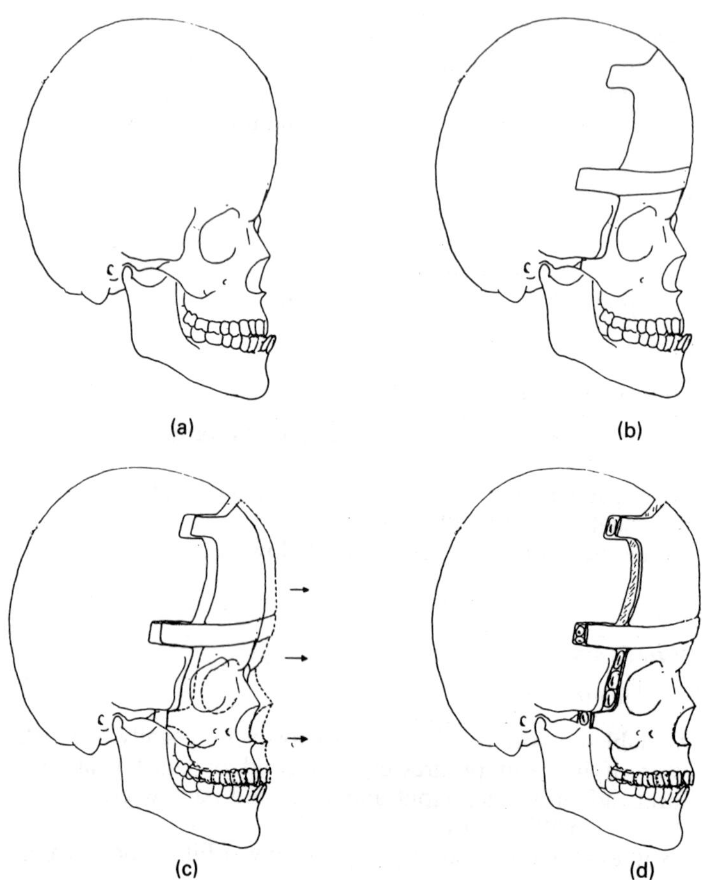

Figure 11.1 Monobloc LeFort III and fronto-orbital advancement for treatment of Crouzon's syndrome. Note that with continued normal growth of the mandible, the patient may require further maxillary advancement surgery at the LeFort I level after the completion of growth. (a) Brachycephalic (steep flat forehead) with total midface retrusion. (b) Outline of osteotomy cuts. (c) Monobloc advancement of midface, orbits and frontal bone. (d) Surgical result – fixation not shown and bone grafting confined to facial skeleton.

Pfeiffer syndrome

Clinical features

1. Turribrachycephaly
2. Hypertelorism – antimongoloid slant, proptosis and strabismus

3. Maxillary hypoplasia – high arched palate, upper dental crowding, facial asymmetry
4. Broad thumbs and great toes – very characteristic
5. Cutaneous syndactyly – of fingers and toes but less severe than Apert's syndrome

Aetiology

Unknown. Autosomal dominant. *Rare* disorder.

Prognosis and treatment

Depending on severity of craniosynostosis, the facial appearance tends to improve with age (see below). Surgical correction of cutaneous syndactyly is undertaken in severe cases.

Surgical treatment of craniosynostosis

Goals of surgery

1. Decompression of the intracranial space to reduce intracranial pressure in order to:

   a. Prevent visual problems
   b. Permit normal mental development

2. Achievement of satisfactory craniofacial form to correct an unusually shaped head so as to:

   a. Promote peer acceptance and normal assimilation into society
   b. Permit normal psychological and behavioural development

Early surgery (undertaken before 1 year of age)

1. Strip craniectomies – best performed before the age of 3 months. Although this technique alone provides adequate intracranial decompression, it does not address the problem of abnormal craniofacial morphology
2. Frontal bone advancement – with or without strip craniectomies, this procedure is the treatment of choice for most craniosynostoses, and is usually performed at 6 months of age
3. Cranial vault remodelling – mainly used as an additional method for reducing vertical height of the cranial vault in patients with turricephaly

4. Craniofacial advancement (monobloc). Where there is severe midface retrusion, respiratory distress, gross exorbitism and corneal exposure, a simultaneous advancement of the forehead, orbits and midface is indicated
5. Shunt surgery. For hydrocephalis, this is preferably done before the craniectomy and cranial vault remodelling

Late surgery (undertaken after 1 year of age)

1. Frontal bone advancement
2. LeFort III osteotomy advancement

   a. Child – there is a current trend for this subcranial osteotomy to be performed in young children to improve respiratory function and craniofacial form before the start of formal schooling
   b. Adult

3. LeFort III osteotomy and frontal bone advancement (*Fig. 11.1*) – this combined procedure involving an intracranial approach with a subcranial osteotomy has a relatively high infection rate
4. Craniofacial advancement (monobloc) – involves advancement of the orbits and midface as one unit but with increased infection rate
5. LeFort II osteotomy advancement – only used in patients with midface hypoplasia and adequate zygomatic projection
6. Orthognathic surgery – in adolescent years, presumably normal mandibular growth will result in a class III dentofacial discrepancy and will necessitate either one- or two-jaw surgery to correct the skeletal base malocclusion

Branchial arch syndromes

Frontonasal dysplasia

Not a well defined syndrome. The facial deformity can range from mild to severe and occurs in variable combinations with other anomalies.

Clinical features

1. Flat broad nasal root
2. *Orbital hypertelorism*

3. Split nares
4. Median cleft lip
5. Epibulbar dermoids – common
6. Radiological features:

    a. Hypoplastic frontal sinuses
    b. Absence of corpus callosum
    c. Hydrocephalus

7. Mental retardation which is present in some patients seems to be directly related to the severity of the hypertelorism

Aetiology and pathogenesis

1. Nasal capsule fails to develop properly and the space normally occupied by the capsule is filled by the primitive brain vesicle resulting in hypertelorism and lack of formation of nasal tip
2. Presently unknown genetic mode of inheritance

Orbital hypertelorism (Fig. 11.2)

Definition. An abnormally wide distance between the orbits. It is not a syndrome but a physical finding associated with other cranial and facial malformations. In telecanthus, only the medial orbital walls are displaced laterally whereas in hypertelorism, the entire orbits and globes are laterally displaced.

Pathological anatomy. Whatever the cause, the principal anatomical abnormality associated with hypertelorism is the increased horizontal width of the anterior part of the ethmoid

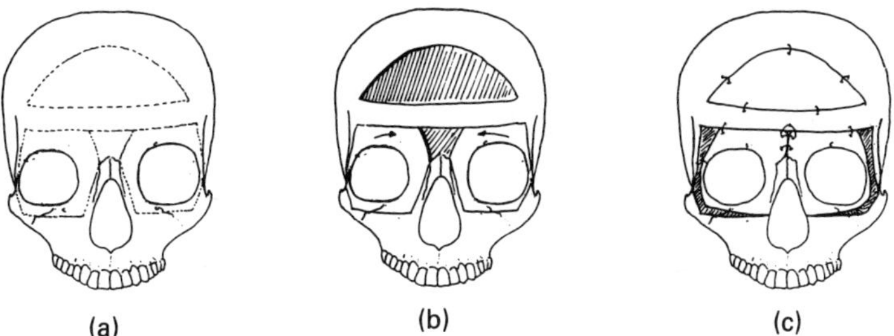

Figure 11.2 Correction of hypertelorism. (a) Osteotomy cuts outlined. (b) Frontal bone flap removed for access to anterior cranial fossa in order to complete cuts across the orbital roof. Portion of ethmoids also removed to permit medial advancement of orbital rims. (c) Surgical result – frontal bone flap replaced as free graft.

sinuses. It was this observation that led to the possibility of surgical correction with preservation of the cribiform plate and olfactory nerves.

Treatment

1. Intracranial approach. Through a frontal craniotomy, the frontal lobes of the brain are raised to expose the osteotomy sites of the anterior cranial fossa. Then the orbital osteotomies are performed and a central segment of ethmoid bone, preserving the cribiform plate, is resected to bring the orbits closer together
2. Extracranial approach. A subcranial procedure alone may be indicated in lesser forms of orbital hypertelorism

Long-term results. Relapse has been noted to occur in some patients, but this was attributed to the degree of the deformity preoperatively rather than the age of the patient at the time of surgery. There is also some evidence that corrective hypertelorism surgery performed in a growing child may interfere with anterior facial growth.

Treacher-collins syndrome (otomandibulofacial dysostosis) (*Fig. 11.3*)

Clinical features

1. Antimongoloid slant of palpebral fissures – coloboma of outer lower eyelid
2. Hypoplastic malars – making nose appear large
3. Micrognathia of mandible – aplastic coronoid and condylar processes; cleft palate in 30% cases
4. Deformed pinna of ear – extra ear tags with blind fistulas may be found anywhere between tragus and angle of mouth
5. Conductive hearing loss
6. Other deformities – absence of parotid gland, congenital heart disease
7. Mental retardation – in some due to hearing deficit

Aetiology and pathogenesis

1. Autosomal dominant – with marked penetrance and variable expressivity

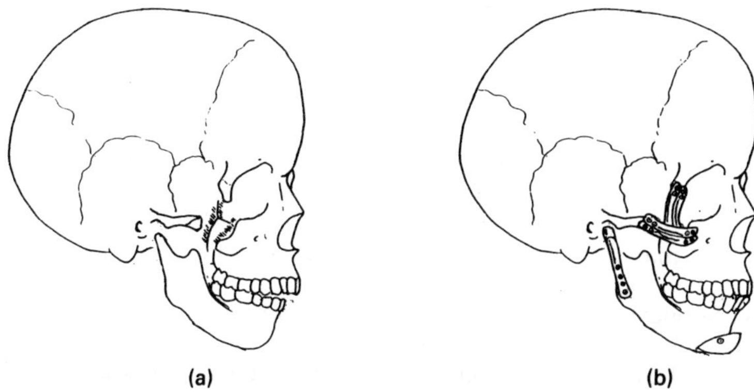

Figure 11.3 Surgical correction of Treacher-Collins syndrome. (a) Note the absent malar complex, mandibular ramus deficiency and anterior open bite. (b) Onlay rib grafts used to reconstruct malar and costochondral rib graft used to reconstruct hypoplastic mandibular condyle as well as advancement genioplasty. Note that where there is a functioning TMJ, it is best to augment mandibular ramus height with inverted 'L' osteotomy.

2. Poswillo (1973) postulates a deformity in the first and second branchial arch due to the death or failure of the preotic neural crest cells to migrate

Differential diagnosis

Acrofacial dysostosis (Nager syndrome). This has a multifactorial inheritance and involves not only the face but also the upper extremities with absent or hypoplastic thumbs, radius, and/or one or more metacarpals; however, similar pathogenesis.

Prognosis

Lifespan not affected unless there are severe cardiac or renal malformations.

Treatment

1. Airway maintenance – severe cases may require tracheostomy
2. Conductive hearing aids – to promote normal speech development
3. Surgical reconstruction of *skeletal deficiencies* – utilizing a

combination of onlay bone grafting with osteotomies to augment the deficiencies in the orbit, malars, maxillae and mandible

a. Orbits and malars – may be grafted in early infancy
b. Maxilla and mandible – usually corrected by orthognathic surgery in adolescence in combination with orthodontic treatment. The main problems are anterior open bite with mandibular retrognathia and microgenia

4. Surgical correction of *soft tissue deformities*

a. Lower eyelid colomboma – corrected with z-plasty
b. Antimongoloid slant of eyelids – hitched up with lateral canthopexy
c. Deformed ears – pose a very difficult reconstructive problem. Recent introduction of implantable ears appears promising

Pierre-Robin syndrome (Pierre Robin anomalad, The Robin sequence)

Clinical features

1. Micrognathia – small mandible which is symmetrically receded. Achieves catch-up growth by 4–6 years old. At birth there is difficulty in inspiratory phase of respiration with periodic cyanotic attacks and laboured breathing
2. Glossoptosis
3. Cleft palate – horse shoe shaped, usually involving soft palate
4. Congenital heart disease – 15–25% of those who die in early infancy
5. Severe mental retardation – 20% cases either primary or secondary to asphyxia

Differential diagnosis

Stickler syndrome may account for as much as 30% of cases of the Robin anomaly.

Aetiology and pathogenesis

1. Does not appear to have a single gene inheritance; may be multifactorial

2. Pathogenesis probably based on arrested development, the primary defect lying in hypoplasia of the mandible preventing the normal descent of the tongue between the palatal shelves
3. A neuromuscular deficiency in the tongue has also been postulated to account for the palatal cleft

Management

Immediate airway maintenance is critical.

1. Keep infant prone with the head pulley-suspended in a stockinette cap
2. Suturing of tip of tongue to lower lip or mandible (temporary)
3. Tracheostomy – in extreme cases
4. *Orthognathic surgery* – depending on the subsequent 'catch-up' growth of the mandible, orthodontics combined with mandibular advancement and genioplasty may be required in later years

Binder's syndrome (nasomaxillary dysplasia)

Clinical features

1. Short nose with absent anterior nasal spine
2. Hypoplastic maxilla – often in the presence of normal malar projection
3. A convex upper lip with an acute nasolabial angle
4. Hypoplastic frontal sinuses

Horswell *et al*. (1988) reviewed 19 patients at the Royal Children's Hospital in Melbourne, Australia and found that patients with Binder's syndrome remain deficient in their horizontal growth (anterior cranial base, horizontal maxilla, nasal projection and columella). However, their vertical growth (maxillary height, nasal and upper lip length), although initially diminished, 'catches up' during the pubertal growth period to normal ranges.

Treatment

1. Perinasal augmentation – onlay grafts as a child
2. Columella lengthening

3. Orthognathic surgical options:

   a. High level (quadrangular) LeFort I maxillary advancement with onlay grafts in the paranasal regions
   b. LeFort II midface advancement – quadrangular, anterior or pyramidal (see Chapter 5)

Other branchial arch syndromes

Craniofacial microsomia

See Chapter 7.

Mobius syndrome

1. Bilateral 6th and 7th nerve palsy
2. High broad nasal bridge
3. Micrognathia – mandible
4. Limb reduction defects and mental deficiency
5. Almost all cases sporadic; rare familial instances
6. Similar pathogenesis to hemifacial microsomia

Hallerman–Streiff syndrome

1. Dyscephaly
2. Micrognathia – anteriorly displaced condyles
3. Hypotrichosis and oligodontia and short stature
4. Congenital cataracts and beaked nose
5. All cases sporadic
6. Pathogenesis – similar to above

Facial clefts

There are over 200 facial cleft syndromes.

1. Oblique facial clefts – may be caused by the failure of covering of the nasolacrimal groove by ectomesenchyme or the result of amniotic bands

   a. Naso-ocular cleft – extending from nostril to lower eyelid border, along the closure of the nasolacrimal groove. Failure of fusion of median nasal, lateral nasal, and maxillary processes

   b. Oro-ocular cleft – extending from eye to lip. Failure of the fused nasal processes to unite with the maxillary nasal process

2. Lateral (transverse) facial cleft – extends from the corner of the mouth to the tragus of the ear. Probably results from incomplete invasion of ectomesenchyme between the maxillary and mandibular parts of the first arch, e.g. macrostomia in hemifacial microsomia patients
3. Cleft lip and/or palate – relatively common (1 in 600) (see Chapter 10)
4. Median cleft of mandible, lower lip and tongue

Further reading

Adus H (1981) Form, function, growth and craniofacial surgery. *Otolaryngol. Clin. North Am.* **14**, 939.

Bachmayer D, Ross B and Munro I (1986) Maxillary growth following LeFort III advancement surgery in Crouzon, Apert and Pfeiffer syndromes. *Am. J. Orthodont.* **90**, 420.

Converse JM, McCarthy JG and Wood-Smith D (1979) Clinical aspects of craniofacial synostosis. In: Converse JM, McCarthy JG, Wood-Smith D (eds): *Symposium on Diagnosis and Treatment of Craniofacial Anomalies.* CV Mosby, St Louis.

Epker BN and Wolford LM (1975) Middle third face osteotomies: their use in the correction of acquired and developmental craniofacial deformities. *J. Oral Surg.* **33**, 491.

Gorlin RJ, Cervenka J and Pruzansky S (1971) Facial clefting and its syndromes. *Birth Defects* **7**, 3.

Gorlin RJ, Cohen MM and Levin LS (1990) *Syndromes of the Head and Neck*. 3rd edn. Oxford University Press, Oxford.

Horswell BB, Holmes AD, Levant BA *et al*. (1988) Cephalometric and anthropomorphic observations of Binder's syndrome: a study of 19 patients. *Plast. Reconstr. Surg.* **81**, 325.

Kaban LB, Conover M and Mulliken JB (1986) Midface position after LeFort III advancement: a long term follow-up study. *Cleft Palate J. Suppl.* **23**, 75.

Kreiborg S and Aduss H (1986) Pre- and postsurgical facial growth in patients with Crouzon's and Apert's syndromes. *Cleft Palate J. Suppl.* **23**, 78.

McCarthy JG (ed) (1990) Cleft lip and palate and craniofacial anomalies. In: *Plastic Surgery* Vol 4, Ch 60–63, pp. 2974–3160. WB Saunders, Philadelphia.

Munro IR (1975) Orbito-cranio-facial surgery: the team approach. *Plast. Reconstr. Surg.* **55**, 170.

Persing JA, Edgerton MT and Jane JA (1989) *Scientific Foundations and Surgical Treatment of Craniosynostosis*. Williams & Wilkins, Baltimore.

Poswillo D (1973) The pathogenesis of the first and second branchial arch syndromes. *Oral Surg.* **35**, 302.

Poswillo D (1974) Orofacial malformations. *Proc. Roy. Soc. Med.* **67**, 343.

Poswillo D (1974) Otomandibular deformity: pathogenesis as a guide to reconstruction. *J. Maxillofac. Surg.* **2**, 64.

Poswillo D (1975) The pathogenesis of Treacher-Collins syndrome (mandibulo-facial dysostosis). *Br. J. Oral Surg.* **13**, 1.
Tessier PJ (1971) Total osteotomy of the middle third of the face for faciostenosis or for sequelae of Le Fort III fractures. *Plast. Reconstr. Surg.* **48**, 533.
Tessier PJ (1971) The definitive plastic surgical treatment of the severe facial deformities of craniofacial dysostosis, Crouzon's and Apert's disease. *Plast. Reconstr. Surg.* **48**, 419.
Tessier PJ (1973) Orbital hypertelorism. *Scand. J. Plast. Surg.* **7**, 39.
Tessier PJ (1976) Anatomical classification of facial, craniofacial and laterofacial clefts. *J. Maxillofac. Surg.* **4**, 69.

Chapter 12

Complications

Introduction

Adverse unplanned events that result in morbity and occasionally mortality. In orthognathic surgery, complications may occur during three distinct phases:

1. Preoperative

Inadequate surgical or orthodontic planning and poor case selection will inevitably trigger complications during the subsequent phases of treatment.

2. Intraoperative

Complications during this phase are often related to poor technique or lack of operator experience. Sometimes it may be the awkward anatomy of the surgical site or difficulties arising from anaesthetic management of the patient that can lead to longer than expected operating time.

3. Postoperative

a. Early – in the days immediately following surgery, complications are usually of an acute nature
b. Late – in the weeks or months after surgery, complications are often of a chronic nature

Complications of mandibular osteotomies

Preoperative phase

1. Patient dissatisfaction – where patient's and/or orthodontist's desires and expectations of treatment differ from the surgeon's

expectations and desires of outcome of treatment. Usually attributed to poor communication between surgeon, orthodontist and patient
2. Errors in diagnosis – and hence inappropriate treatment planning
3. Errors in bite registration – due to inability to achieve centric relation, hence plaster models are mounted incorrectly
4. Surgical occlusal wafers – poorly constructed or made to incorrect jaw relationships
5. Poor patient–doctor rapport
6. Patient is a poor surgical risk for lengthy elective procedures – severely compromised medical status which is not recognized by the clinician

Intraoperative phase

1. *Sagittal split ramus osteotomy*

   a. Unfavourable osteotomy split – especially in the presence of impacted lower third molars or unusual mandibular morphology

      - Buccal plate fracture
      - Inferior alveolar nerve trapped in proximal segment
      - Lingual plate fracture of distal segment
      - Horizontal fracture of ascending ramus
      - Fracture of condylar process

   b. Nerve injury

      - Inferior alveolar nerve – may be stretched, avulsed, torn or compressed during the split, manipulation and fixation of the proximal and distal segments
      - Facial nerve – rare, but may occur in large mandibular set-backs where the medial cut is extended to the posterior border of ascending ramus

   c. Haemorrhage – occasionally the inferior alveolar artery, retromandibular veins and rarely the facial and maxillary vessels may be a source of troublesome bleeding
   d. Malposition of proximal segment

      - Counterclockwise rotation

- Condylar distraction or malposition in posterior, anterior or lateral direction

2. *Vertical subsigmoid ramus osteotomy*

   a. Unfavourable osteotomy

      - Subcondylar rather than lower border

   b. Nerve Injury – inferior alveolar nerve

      - Excessive medial dissection of soft tissues
      - Medial displacement of mobile proximal segment
      - Bone cut made too far forward

   c. Haemorrhage

      - Maxillary artery
      - Inferior alveolar artery

   d. Proximal segment malposition

      - Condylar sag
      - Medial or posterior displacement

3. *Mandibular body osteotomies*

   a. Unfavourable osteotomy
   b. Nerve injury
   c. Haemorrhage
   d. Malpositioning of mobilized segments
   e. Damage to teeth
   f. Vascular compromise – stretching or tearing of the vascular pedicle may significantly compromise postoperative healing

Postoperative phase

1. *Relapse*

   Important influencial factors

   - Suprahyoid musculature and investing soft tissues
   - Type of fixation

- Magnitude of mandibular advancement
- Area of bony contact at osteotomy site
- Condylar distraction and position of proximal fragment

Mandibular advancements

- The greater the mandibular advancement, the greater the magnitude of relapse which occurs
- Rigid internal fixation has resulted in increased stability for small to moderate advancements but appears to have less influence on large advancements (i.e. > 6 mm)
- Suprahyoid myotomy has been shown to increase stability in primates but not shown in humans
- Questionable whether increase in posterior facial height necessarily increases the chance of relapse

Mandibular set-back

- Relapse tends to occur in growing patients
- May occur with rotation of the proximal segment
- In non-growing patients, however, it is a relatively stable operation with some posterior movement postoperatively
- This seems to be the only operation in which rigid fixation may not play a necessary role

2. Neurological dysfunction

The chances of mental nerve dysfunction are more likely with:

a. Sagittal split ramus osteotomy
b. Older patients > 40 years
c. Simultaneous genioplasty

3. Mandibular dysfunction

a. Hypomobility with reduced mandibular opening
b. Reduction in bite force
c. Temporomandibular joint dysfunction

  - Myofascial pain
  - Joint arthrosis
  - Condylar resorption

d. Malocclusion either due to relapse or poor intraoperative dental positioning

4. Other

a. Secondary haemorrhage
b. Infection
c. Malunion, delayed union, non-union
d. Wound dehiscence
e. Poor aesthetics – i.e. double chining created by mandibular set-back

Complications of maxillary surgery

Preoperative complications

Essentially similar to those of mandibular osteotomies (see above).

Intraoperative complications

1. Unfavourable osteotomy

a. Horizontal fracture of pterygoid plates
b. High horizontal fracture of pyramidal process of palatine bone
c. Fracture at the junction of horizontal process of palatine bone with palatal process of maxilla

2. Haemorrhage

Vessels of greatest concern are:

a. Maxillary artery and its terminal branches
b. Descending palatine arteries
c. Pterygoid venous plexus
d. Internal carotid artery – rare

Note: Hypotensive anaesthesia has enabled minimal blood loss in LeFort I downfracture procedures.

3. Improper maxillary positioning

a. Bony or soft tissue interferences, i.e. inadequate ostectomies
b. Inadequate surgical reference points
c. Inadequate mobilization of maxilla

4. Inability to stabilize maxilla

Due to inadequate bone contact at osteotomy sites. Best to use rigid fixation and if gaps are wide enough, then interpositional bone grafting may be warranted.

5. Other

a. Prolapse of buccal fat pad
b. Perforation of nasoendotracheal tube
c. Damage to teeth

- Segmental osteotomies
- Low osteotomy cut

d. Oronasal communication

- maxillary expansion

e. Buckled nasal septum – maxillary impaction without adequate septal trimming

Postoperative complications

1. Relapse

Cause

a. Growing patient
b. Lack of complete mobilization before repositioning
c. Insufficient bone union – poor bone contact or no bone grafts used
d. Inadequate fixation

Prevention

a. Good case selection and proper treatment planning. (i.e. good presurgical orthodontics)
b. Effective bone grafting

c. Slight overcorrection
d. Adequate fixation

Relapse characteristics (Welch 1989)

a. Maxillary impaction – tends to be a stable operation, and what relapse does occur will generally be in the superior direction. Bimaxillary surgery, with mandibular advancement, appears to be more stable than with single jaw alone, requiring maxillary impaction
b. Maxillary downgraft – has a tendency to be unstable with relapse occurring in a variety of directions, especially upward and backwards. The upper lip has a tendency to lengthen postoperatively. Currently, there is no way to predict which patients will have a tendency to relapse and in what direction it will occur
c. Maxillary advancement – tends to be a stable operation but there is some degree of upper lip retraction that occurs postoperatively. What magnitude of advancement requires bone grafts for stability is still undetermined
d. Lefort III osteotomy – appears to be a stable procedure in non-growing patients
e. Cleft palate patients – LeFort I osteotomy tends to be an unstable procedure in these patients with unique problems such as inadequate mobilization due to scarring, but some are similar to problems in normal patients with vertical maxillary deficiency

Note: There are often problems in interpreting results because of problems with design of studies and the multifactorial nature of the problem.

2. Haemorrhage

Postoperative haemorrhage after LeFort I osteotomy.

Sources of bleeding

a. Internal maxillary artery – most vulnerable at the pterygopalatine fossa when osteotome is used at the pterygoid plates
b. Greater palatine artery – usually seen and controlled intraoperatively
c. Pterygoid plexus – venous bleeding on downfracture
d. Internal carotid artery and internal jugular vein – rarely

Clinical presentation

a. Anterior epistaxis – bleeding from nose
b. Posterior epistaxis – bleeding backwards into mouth or pharynx
c. Anxiety and shock

Suggested management protocol

a. Rapid release of MMF and clearing of oral, nasal and pharyngeal clots to locate bleeding source
b. Admission for observation, bedrest and sedation – if minor bleeding
c. Monitor vital signs – estimate blood loss, order full blood examination, coagulation studies, cross-match blood. IV fluid replacement, plasma expanders or blood replacement
d. Insertion of Foley catheter to posterior nasal space which is then replaced by anterior and posterior nasal packs which may be left *in situ* for 2–4 days
e. Tracheostomy – should be considered if airway is in jeopardy
f. Surgical exposure of maxillary sinus by redownfracture and inserting a pack (Surgicel or Avitene) for 7–10 days or location and clipping of suspected vessels, i.e. posterior nasal, sphenopalatine and descending palatine arteries, at the back of the maxilla
g. Ligation of external carotid artery or more proximal branches of internal maxillary artery – may be ineffective because of anastomosing branches derived from different sources
h. Angiography and embolization – of distal branches of maxillary artery.

   Technique – catheter is passed under fluoroscopic control from femoral artery at the groin, to the aortic arch, common carotid, external carotid and then selectively into internal maxillary artery. Embolization is achieved by pieces of Gelfoam delivered to bleeding site via catheter.
   New technique – transcatheter electrocoagulation, still being refined before routine use

3. Neurological dysfunction

Commonly neuropraxia injury to infraorbital nerve (V2). However, injury to the abducens nerve and parasympathetic fibres of lacrimal gland have been reported. The latter injuries have been purported to arise from awkward pterygomaxillary dysjunction

4. Unfavourable facial aesthetics

Particularly the soft tissue changes in the nasolabial region. Undesirable changes which can occur as a result of maxillary surgery include:

a. Widening of alar bases
b. Increased prominence of alar groove
c. Upturning of nasal tip
d. Shortening and thinning of upper lip

5. Infection

a. Free bone sequestra
b. Emphysema in cheeks – noseblowing
c. Maxillary sinus problems
d. Loose fixation
e. Wound dehiscence

6. Tooth vitality

In animal studies, degenerative pulpal changes after LeFort I osteotomies have been observed as a result of transient pulpal vascular ischaemia and direct injury to apices of teeth.

Di *et al*. 1988 (Dallas, Texas) observed that the LeFort I downfracture had little discernible effect on the pulp and on the development of human third molar teeth that were extracted after maxillary osteotomy.

7. Other

a. Velopharyngeal incompetence – with large maxillary advancements
b. Oronasal fistula – width excessive midpalatal expansion. Best to use paramedian palatal osteotomies where palatal thickness is much greater, i.e. horseshoe

Further reading

Carlotti AE and Schendel SA (1987) An analysis of factors influencing the stability of surgical advancement of the maxilla by the LeFort I osteotomy. *J. Oral Maxillofac. Surg.* **45**, 924.

Carlson DS, Ellis III EE and Dechow PC (1987) Adaptation of the suprahyoid muscle complex to mandibular advancement surgery. *Am. J. Orthod. Dentofac. Orthop.* **92**, 134.

Di S, Bell WH, Mannai C *et al*. (1988) Long term evaluation of teeth after LeFort I osteotomy: a histologic and developmental study. *Oral Surg. Oral Med. Oral Pathol.* **65**, 379.

Epker BN and La Banc JP (1990) Orthognathic surgery: management of post-operative complications. *Oral Maxillofac. Surg. Clin. North Am.* **2**, 901.

Franco JE, Van Sickels JE and Thrash WJ (1989) Factors contributing to relapse in rigidly fixed mandibular setbacks. *J. Oral Maxillofac. Surg.* **47**, 451.

Lanigan DT and West RA (1984) Management of post-operative haemorrhage following the LeFort I maxillary osteotomy. *J. Maxillofac. Surg.* **42**, 367.

Lanigan DT (1990) Haemorrhage associated with orthognathic surgery. *Oral. Maxillofac. Surg. Clin. North Am.* **2**, 887.

Martis CS (1984) Complications after mandibular sagittal split osteotomy. *J. Oral Maxillofac. Surg.* **42**, 101.

O'Ryan F (1990) Complications of orthognathic surgery. *Oral Maxillofac. Surg. Clin. North Am.* **2**, 593.

Sinn DP and Ghali GE (1990) Management of intraoperative complications in orthognathic surgery. *Oral Maxillofac. Surg. Clin. North Am.* **2**, 869.

Tuinzing DB and Greebe RB (1985) Complications related to the intraoral vertical ramus osteotomy. *Int. J. Oral Surg.* **14**, 319.

Turvey T (1985) Intraoperative complications of sagittal osteotomy of the mandibular ramus: incidence and management. *J. Oral Maxillofac. Surg.* **43**, 504.

Van Sickels JE, Larsen AJ and Thrash WJ (1986) Relapse after rigid fixation of mandibular advancement. *J. Oral Maxillofac. Surg.* **44**, 698.

Welch TB (1989) Stability in the correction of dentofacial deformities: a comprehensive review. *J. Oral Maxillofac. Surg.* **47**, 1142.

Will LA, Joondeph DR, Hohl TH *et al*. (1984) Condylar position following mandibular advancement: its relationship to relapse. *J. Oral Maxillofac. Surg.* **42**, 578.

Index